Fit Feet for Life

To my three children Luis, Cruz, and Elia.

Acknowledgments

I would like to thank the people without whom this book would not have happened.

Many thanks to:
Philip and Felix Artzt, Anne Telahr, Werner Kieser, Dr. Homayun Gharavi, Wolf Harwarth, Christoph Limberger, Mira Hampel, Marius Keckeisen, and five Konzept, Inc.

Marco Montanez

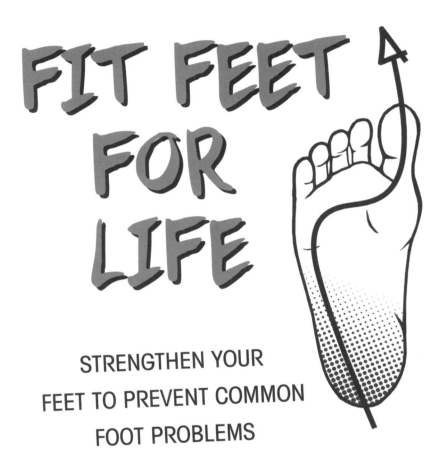

FIT FEET FOR LIFE

STRENGTHEN YOUR FEET TO PREVENT COMMON FOOT PROBLEMS

MEYER & MEYER SPORT

British Library Cataloguing in Publication Data
A catalogue record for this book is available from the British Library

Originally published as *Unfuck Your Feet*, © 2018 by Meyer & Meyer Verlag

Fit Feet for Life
Maidenhead: Meyer & Meyer Sport (UK) Ltd., 2020
ISBN: 978-1-78255-183-6

© 2020 by Meyer & Meyer Sport (UK) Ltd.
Aachen, Auckland, Beirut, Dubai, Hägendorf, Hong Kong, Indianapolis, Cairo, Cape Town, Manila, Maidenhead, New Delhi, Singapore, Sydney, Tehran, Vienna
🖎 Member of the World Sports Publishers' Association (WSPA),
   www.w-s-p-a.org
Printed by C-M Books, Ann Arbor, MI
ISBN: 978-1-78255-183-6
Email: info@m-m-sports.com
www.thesportspublisher.com

CONTENTS

PREFACE
BY WERNER KIESER

Thank you so much! This book is needed – meaning, it meets a need.

This need is not yet fully appreciated by the experts, not to mention the "foot folk" in the truest sense of the word. I became aware of my ignorance on this subject through a personal experience.

I had suffered for years from a recurring pain in the little toe of my left foot. On our travels, my wife and I often find ourselves walking for hours and hours through the cities that we visit. Nine years ago in Berlin, the pain in my toe was present as usual, therefore diminishing the pleasure of a city walk. "Look, they have barefoot shoes. Why don't you buy a pair?" asked my (physician) wife as we stood in front of a shoe store. Somewhat reluctant and rather acquiescent, I tried on a few different models and ended up purchasing a pair. I wore the new shoes out of the store and for the duration of our continued hike.

The result was shocking. The pain in my little toe disappeared within the hour (although it felt more like a minute). It was in fact gone forever which made me wonder...As a strength trainer, I should have paid much more attention to the subject of "feet." To close this gap, I not only immersed myself in the biomechanics of the foot, but also in its evolution. I acquired footprints of our closest relatives (gorillas, chimpanzees, orangutans). Whenever visitors to my library discover these specimens, they ask: "are those ape hands?" No, they are feet that look like our hands.

And it was then that it dawned on me: our feet are also primarily prehensile organs, suitable for walking but not running. This is something that would require hoofs, but we are not running animals. When I voiced and explained my opinion during a newspaper interview, I experienced what today would be called a *shit-storm*. I had clearly touched a nerve.

This harsh reaction motivated me to research this subject within a societal context. I considered two factors as plausible: first, a multi-billion dollar industry postulates that jogging is sacrosanct and totally healthy as long as you have the right running shoes that unburden, cushion, and support the feet – and cost a fortune. The fact that the foot itself is the best running shoe and is weakened by this girdle is ignored and concealed.

Secondly, I observed obvious addictive behavior among serious runners in my circle of friends and acquaintances, triggered by a daily endorphin release. This also explained the irrational reactions to my doubts about the purpose of jogging. If we were to permanently treat our hands like feet, there would be no pianists in the world. I congratulate the author on his courage and hope that this book reaches readers around the world.

Werner Kieser

PREFACE
BY DR. HOMAYUN GHARAVI

An awesome book! Educational and inspirational for everyone!

We have made many things in life easier with advancements in medicine and technology, but we certainly haven't made all of them healthier. The reason is the fact that medicine is fundamentally pathology-oriented. This means that during our training, we physicians study all of the pathological deviations from the normal state, but not the way we can move from a non-pathological starting point to an even healthier state. The science of health, salutology, is still dismissed. Meanwhile, many pathological conditions are developing beneath our healthy façade that will only become apparent some time in the future.

Let's assume we see a doctor while we are healthy, and to the question: "what ails you today?" we reply with: "nothing at all, Doctor. But what can I do to keep it this way?" The doctor would have to take some time to talk to us about our lifestyle and then eventually offer advice on improvements that could be made in order to ensure our health. These lines make even me laugh out loud. It is a physical impossibility!

All too often, technological progress has taken a wrong turn and built an impressive building in the wrong spot. In the case of footwear, modern shoe technology is the result of an initial mistake, separating the person from contact with the earth via a cushion. What has followed is a chain-reaction of unwanted side effects and their counter-measures. The modern shoe has ended up at the end of the longest chain-reaction.

With this work, Marco Montanez, who has never been afraid of detours in his life when it comes to acquiring a downright incomparable wealth of experience in many different areas, has delivered a true masterpiece.

He manages to make a complex topic easily digestible and entertaining with plain language. I am sure that even physicians and physical therapists will gain many valuable concepts and examples for explanatory approaches as I have, that will give new impetus to their work with patients. Because the shoe is not a natural habitat for our feet.

Fit Feet for Life – a long overdue emergency guide for your feet.

Unf*ck your feet – and you will experience movement in a whole new way.

Dr. Homayun Gharavi

1 UNF*CK YOUR FEET!

According to the dictionary, *unfuck* is a colloquialism for solving a mistake or a problem.

Unfuck your feet is a clear statement, an announcement and appeal, based on evolution, the laws of nature, and not least of all common sense. It is an exciting change of perspective and a review of well-known wisdoms about all things feet. We dispel dangerous superficial knowledge, present facts and use logic as we take a look at human locomotion and its offshoots, such as jogging, Nordic walking, and the forefoot strike, from an evolutionary point of view without getting overly intellectual or trying to impress with medical and sports-scientific terminology.

It is about reviewing habits and knowing the difference between normal and natural. The *unfuck* principle can be applied to the feet as well as many other areas of life.

It is a development like we have seen for many years now in the area of nutrition. Just like some people put Chia seeds in their Paleo cereal or drink green smoothies by the gallon, there are those for whom Diet Coke and a donut are a permanent fixture of their diet. It may be normal, but it certainly isn't natural.

"If walking barefoot is only a trend, it has been trending for the past two million years and will continue to prevail in the future."

Dr. Daniel Lieberman, Harvard University

Hardly any other body part is so blatantly neglected. And we're not talking about purely esthetic aspects like polishing your toenails or removing calluses. It is a fundamental problem, and the subject of feet is a subject that elicits very different reactions in people.

People's ambivalent relationship with their feet is apparent in the almost contemptuous conditions that we keep them in and expect them to put up with. Sadly, we take better care of our pets than ourselves, so it doesn't come as a surprise that we cripple ourselves with misinterpreted and fashion-inspired footwear. We would never put shoes on our pets, our cats and dogs, because not only would it look silly, but it would also restrict their movement ability to such an extent that their natural desire to move would not only be impaired, but completely inhibited. However, the animals' adaptability would allow them to get used to it, and the initially unsound movement patterns would gradually change to clumping and finally to an increasingly better coordinated movement that still would not look natural, but at some point would at least be considered normal. However, this does not conform to nature.

This is similar to insight such as knowing that excessive drinking of cow's milk is normal, but not natural. While it is an intolerance most of us possess, like with gluten or lactose, there are also people with different tolerances to plastic foam. Some may tolerate it more than others. This book, however, is a way out of rubber foam intolerance.

The following pages are the result of my intensive engagement in recent years with the theory and science surrounding the feet and their practical application in the form of species-appropriate locomotion. Next to countless studies, it primarily reflects the experience and feedback from hundreds of people I have coached or trained, and from thousands who have listened to my lectures.

If the effect that my coaching and lectures has on people could be multiplied rudimentarily, it would make a significant difference. If nothing else, this book is also for all the people that were at first curious, then astonished, and finally shocked by the truths imparted on them, but also for those who have not yet attended one of my lectures. I do have to admit that before the start of every lecture, I always feel like this is something that everyone should know by now, and am still surprised when this is disproven.

"Research means seeing what everyone else sees, and thinking what no one else has thought before."

Albert Szent-Gyorgyi

2 STRENGTH FROM THE EARTH

In the fall of 2012, I had a life-changing and mind-blowing experience. I was working out alone with my Wing Tsun instructor and as was so often the case, it was about using two of the principles of power of the intelligent Chinese martial arts system in which everything is about movement efficiency and optimization.

To me "Give up your own force!" And "Make your opponent give up his force!" was as logical as practically applicable in theory and in practice. But when training with my instructor, I was far from movement efficiency and optimization, and giving up my own force and that of my teacher merely consisted in clumsily finding my balance and falling off of the balance beam.

Only now, after years of intensive study, did I receive the critical advice in an accessory sentence.

"Take off your shoes!"

This was such simple advice that it initially caused me to hesitate and wonder if I was wearing clean socks. I thought about whether I should open the window before taking off my shoes. I stood on the balance beam, a wooden structure shaped like the letter H, on which one can stand and practice with a partner. Having regained their freedom, my feet activated their muscular and proprioceptive potential and clutched the approx. 10 cm wide and 5 cm deep wooden beam. My big toe literally gripped the edge and my ankle worked to keep me upright, restoring my balance instead of further leaving that job to my all too frantically working hips. This momentous experience was very brief, since coordinating these new abilities took lots of effort. I lacked strength, but that brief phase during which my body functioned as one unit from the bottom up, had whetted my appetite for more.

Overwhelmed by this experience, I got online and searched for options to avoid training in my socks or barefoot and wear as minimal a shoe as possible. The choice of products was slim and did not meet my criteria. That is when I ordered my first pair of *barefoot shoes*. Spurred on by the experience, they replaced my usual footwear from that day forward. While playing tennis, during strength training and Wing Tsun, and especially in my daily life, I now moved almost barefoot.

My awareness of the surface on which I moved had changed. With every step, my expanded awareness of the ground provided me with new and sometimes intense experiences. Paving stones, cobbles, or gravel paths made every step an adventure and my soles did not just became more perceptive and adaptable, but also stronger.

The change was particularly pronounced on the tennis court. I was literally lighter on my feet while loosely hitting the ball with students, which seemed extraordinary to me. Liberated from those massive plastic foam wedges, I used my feet much more consciously and my legs more quickly. I initially lacked control and strength during extreme movements like, for instance, sliding to the ball or sudden directional changes. But it was astonishing how quickly my feet adjusted and how efficiently I was able to move, for example from one corner of the court back to the center, when I worked with my legs directly on the ground. I could feel the court. It felt good right from the start and those eight hours on the tennis court that usually meant tired, painful feet were now a thing of the past.

I occasionally even forgot to take them off unlike normally, when I took off my tightly-laced tennis shoes as fast as possible, removed my socks and released my soggy and deformed feet into flip-flops. By the way, my shoes got lots of attention and the reactions varied. There was incomprehension of how I could wear them to play tennis, and ridicule because the front of my shoes were so wide that they looked like flippers. I took in every comment and question and devised responses, verbal and athletic, whereby I gave some on the spot and demonstrated that it wasn't my shoes that performed, but my feet.

My training increasingly changed and I also integrated my insights into my teaching. Biomechanics and efficient movement have always been pillars of my teaching method, and I was fascinated at how well my mostly adolescent students adjusted.

When they took off their shoes during training, their stride frequency, directional changes, and posture automatically changed. What I had previously only been able to achieve more or less well with instruction, they now instinctively did right as they reacted to their newfound strength from the ground.

A young female student had regularly complained about pain in the heel and Achilles tendon. After a visit to the orthopedist, she began to train with the prescribed orthotic that raised the heel and initially allowed her to train pain-free. Delighted with the solution to her problem, she was back to diligent training, but then started to experience problems with ankle stability. While the orthotic had relieved the tightness in the Achilles tendon by lifting the heel, that lift had also raised the center of gravity and changed the body tension. This in turn amplified the leverage effect of the raised shoe sole and resulted in some strange situations.

I suggested that she remove the orthotic, and after consulting her mother we went back to training barefoot. The pain then went away and the stability visibly increased. This result initially contradicted everything I had learned and experienced over the past 25 years. If such minor changes to the foundation could have such major effects, it was something that would have to be known. However, aside from the usual orthopedic lunacy like orthotics and bandages, there was nothing that would even begin to support or explain what I had experienced.

When I was young, I also played tennis with bandages and supports after rolling my ankle several times. In basketball for instance, tightly laced high-tops were a must. In Munich, I regularly trained with the Bavarian Tennis Association's youth players at the Sport-Scheck all-weather facility, a large beautifully situated, multi-functional tennis and fitness complex. The age of the boys and girls ranged from nine to twelve years old, and they were already so conditioned that they weren't ready to play until after they had put on their ankle brace or athletic tape. Even the men's national league players on the world-ranking list at the Rochus Club did not hit a ball until they had donned their bandages and braces. The insecurity and dependency was so extreme that it was no longer possible to train without an ankle brace. And in spite of bandages, orthotics, and athletic tape, or maybe because of these things, the players were regularly complaining of pain.

I contacted the manufacturer of my barefoot shoes to seek cooperation. I wanted to obtain shoes for my clients and myself and share my experience with barefoot shoes as a training tool. After lots of meetings and conversations, we agreed to collaborate and came up with a concept for fitness studios to sell shoes in the future. During a promotional tour, we visited the "Rückgrat" in Donaueschingen where I met the owner Lutz Kruger and the physical therapist Wolf Harwath. At that time, they introduced me to their Five concept. On the top floor were pieces of wooden furniture, apparently placed there for the fitness studio members. Five, the movement concept, consisted of wooden pieces of equipment with which one could primarily achieve what seemed like an uncomfortable backwards movement.

Some of the movements seemed familiar since I had completed the *Chikung* training during my Wing Tsun instructor training at my association of the European Wing Tsun organization. This concept is based on traditional Chinese Qigong, but, as I only learned a few years ago, was heavily influenced by Walter Packi's biokinematics. Sifu Roland Liebscher-Bracht, who now has successfully adopted and refined many of the approaches with his LNB method, facilitated the training.

One thing I particularly liked was the fact that you had to take off your shoes before you could start with the training. On that particular day it was very busy, and I watched as one member after another took off his shoes without objection in order to start the training.

One implement roused my curiosity. Next to the handrail was a wooden plank equipped with wooden dowels and three structures resembling a coupling device. Lutz explained that it was a dummy, a first trial version that was being tested here at "Rückgrat" for its applicability. The feedback must have been pretty good because when I returned to "Rückgrat" a few months later for my first barefoot running workshop, a full-size version, the *five feet*, stood in front of the entrance of the spinning room.

During the first training clinic with Lee Saxby in Germany that was held at "Rückgrat," I assisted the biomechanics expert and "Born to Run" coach. After the three-day seminar, I became the first barefoot coach in Germany to be certified by him and the famous Harvard professor Dr. Daniel Lieberman. I subsequently went on to train the majority of the numerous barefoot trainers in Germany.

During that time, I became keenly aware of two things. First, how far-reaching and important the knowledge imparted in my workshops really was. And secondly, how difficult it is to implement these really quite simple truths.

One of my tennis students asked me one day after practice if I could talk to his co-workers about feet. In the course of the conversation, we agreed to collaborate with Kieser Training AG, and I developed a training concept that focused on training the feet based on the hierarchy of human locomotion, standing, walking, and running. With emphasis on the essential: *Unfuck your Feet.*

3 IF THE SHOE FITS

It comes as no surprise, but when I think about it, I have always worn shoes. As a child, I wore slippers so my feet wouldn't get cold. Right after getting out of bed I was told: "Put on your slippers!" It was a well-intended, increasingly insistent plea by my mother. I always had to wear slippers so I wouldn't catch a cold.

I have worn many shoes for different purposes and occasions and somehow they all had one thing in common. At first they felt funny on my feet although they had a great insole. But they somehow never seemed to fit, and if you have children you know that kids think shoes are stupid unless they blink or have a Spiderman design. In my case, the sales clerk was always reassuring and promising my mother and me that regular wear would make the shoes even softer and more comfortable. I remember it very well, because my feet weren't normal but very wide with a high instep. This was confirmed during a visit to a trusted shoe store, and with feet this wide, it just wasn't easy to find shoes that fit.

We ultimately found some that fit, and in the future it was the eye and not the foot that decided which model should be worn. The feet had to abide by the decision, but sometimes they seemed to fight the shoe, namely when seams would come apart, soles would wear unevenly, or the lining would be pushed through, particularly where the big toe resided.

Later on there were fancy leather shoes from a major Italian fashion designer, which I still own today, stored in a nice bag with a shoe stretcher. The last time I wore them was at a conference where the dress code dictated a black suit, and I wished to wear the appropriate attire. I changed from barefoot to leather wedges in the parking garage, which I almost immediately regretted because my feet acknowledged the unfamiliar tightness and slant with massive pain. During the short walk to the stairwell, I felt so "disabled" by the shoes that I limped back to my car and changed shoes.

There was and is the proper shoe for every occasion, which recently led me to slip on my soccer shoes. I put them on for my children who had found my old soccer shoes in the basement and brought them up into the light of day. Just lacing the shoes was so unpleasant that I only tied them in a loose bow instead of the normally tight laces. After a few minutes, I understood why soccer players always lie on the ground for such a long time after they're fouled, because those things were barely tolerable even while lying down.

"I have no special talent, I am just passionately curious."

Albert Einstein

4 EVOLUTIONARY MASTERPIECE

The feet are a unique feature of the human being. This evolutionary masterpiece consists of approx. 26 bones, 33 joints, and 60 muscles. More than 100 ligaments and many tendons form a transverse and longitudinal arch. They carry the weight of the body, buffer blows, and transmit power. Receptors on the soles signal information about the ground's properties and our position in space to our spinal cord and brain. This allows our central nervous system to control our movements in a natural, healthy, and efficient way.

We spend hours on them. The first thing we do in the morning is stand up, and they do their job, usually unconsciously and unnoticed. They are the foundation, our base. We stand our ground when we must, and when we are sick and not doing well, we want to quickly get back on our feet so we can have both feet on the ground again. We want to gain a foothold in a new area, and we like to say that the shoemaker's son always goes barefoot.

The first thing we want to learn as children and forget as adults is the ability to move under our own steam. In stark contrast to this is the number of pedestrians who can only walk with walkers, orthopedic footwear, or not at all. More than half of all people in industrial nations suffer from foot problems.

The proof is alarming. 98% of infants are born with healthy feet. But only one third don't have problems with their feet as adults. Nearly six million Germans suffer from "hallux valgus," the crooked big toe that is still dismissed as a congenital disorder instead of acknowledging the fact that there is no hallux-valgus gene. Tests done on school-aged children show that 12% of preschoolers and elementary school students already show signs of foot damage. That foot damage increases and worsens with age. Experts estimate that 80% of Germans have problems with their feet. The most common conditions are an enlarged ball of the foot, hammertoe, corns, fallen arches, and splayfoot.

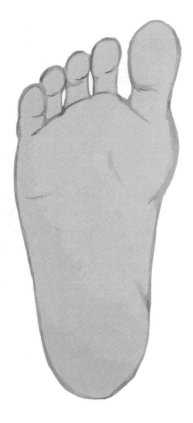

Fig. 1: The human foot

5 FOOTLOOSE

The significance and perception of the feet varies in different cultures. For example, the washing of feet in the Christian faith symbolizes the cleansing from head to toe. An Islamic place of worship can only be entered in bare feet because only the foot creates the connection with and rootedness to the earth. In China, the feet of privileged women were systematically crippled until the early 20th century. Girls as young as six or seven had their toes bound under their feet to achieve an ideal size of 7.5 cm (3 inches). It is the origin of the *lotus feet*, whose shape symbolized the vagina and was considered particularly erotic.

The affected women were unable to move on their unbound, literally "free feet," just like the naked feet of slaves, who were forbidden to wear shoes as a clear sign of dependence and subjugation. Their masters wore shoes with heels as ladies and gentlemen have done in different eras, to emphasize their position and set themselves apart from the common folk.

It is no secret, and one must not have a degree in sports science to know that regular exercise is the foundation to a healthy life. In spite of, or maybe because it is so obvious, modern humans reject the idea even though exercise is the most powerful antidote to diseases of civilization and modern epidemics like diabetes, cancer, heart ailments, and depression.

The range of suitable exercise opportunities is more than enough, thanks to the constantly growing fitness industry and its diverse offerings.

Regardless of the type of exercises that we engage in, or which fitness studio offering we choose from such as Zumba and circuit training, all the way to CrossFit and functional training, everything is based on our natural ability to stand, walk, and run. No matter what or how we move, every movement, every sport, every workout is based on the perfect functioning of our feet.

But why do people increasingly lose the ability to move under their own steam? Why do we get injured when we do what is good for us, and in spite of having access to increasingly better supporting technologies? Better shock absorption, more intelligent foam materials for efficient energy retrieval, and sophisticated support and control mechanisms should not only make us faster and give us more endurance, but also protect us from injury. The reason is simple. We have forgotten how to stand, walk, and run.

6 MARKETING OR EVOLUTION?

Natural running or barefoot running has been a topic that to date has been covered in countless reports and commentaries, not least because of the bestseller *Born to Run*.

Next to the certainly thrilling experience of feeling Mother Earth again, or some idealists who walk barefoot across cars in protest, there is also the orthotics and the esthetic theory of chiropody. Recommendations for barefoot running from orthopedists are limited because they don't actually mean running, but instead walking. They only suggest walking without socks and shoes at home. Orthodox medical practitioners, physical therapists, and orthopedists say that barefoot running is healthy, but only in moderation and not for everyone, thereby acknowledging the health benefits of barefoot walking and running only to immediately misuse them and sell orthotics, wraps, and surgeries.

Even if the logic of reduction and a return to our innate abilities make lots of sense, the influence of industry and the marketing machine that has penetrated us from earliest childhood with its dangerous slogans and promises, is too great for us to accept this stunningly simple solution to this plight. The human brain isn't as easily sealed off or switched to the factory setting as we are accustomed to from our electronic devices. We also don't possess a built-in "bullshit filter," and information is gathered all the time and everywhere, being stored without thinking or consenting.

In the same way that milk products, peanut butter, and orange juice are a normal part of our diets in order to cover our daily requirement of calcium, vitamins and other nutrients from dairy, so is the trip to our trusted sporting goods store when we want to start running again. Every spring, usually even right after Christmas when sugar and wheat consumption have peaked, it is time to eat humble pie. During this quest, the good intentions are channeled into replacing the once again too tight workout clothes and worn out running shoes, leading most people to the nearest sporting goods store. The result is that they leave the store as over-pronators and $200 lighter, but with awesome cushioning, anti-pronation support, and varying spring, lift, and arch.

To understand what went wrong, let's take a look at our evolutionary history. There are still people who ignore Darwin's theory of evolution and pronounce us as God's creation. Even though I value and have read the Bible, I would nevertheless like to refer to all of the scientific evidence regarding our origin.

These studies confirm that our body in all of its relevant biomechanical functions resembles that of the hunter-gatherer from 200,000 years ago, and the ability to run long distances upright was one, if not the most important, factor in our evolution as the most dominant species on our planet.

This evolutionary competitive edge allowed us to cover long distances with a high degree of energy efficiency – usually barefoot. The large prey we ran down served as a source of protein for our growing brain and provided the foundation for the exodus from East Africa into the entire world – wholly without running shoes.

7 A BIG STEP FOR MANKIND

Without running shoes, and in the beginning definitely without any kind of footwear, human evolution was a process that spanned several million years and took place under some severe geological and climactic influences. We would not exist in our current form had it not been for the many climate leaps during the quaternary ice age, the most recent period of earth's history that started 2.6 million years ago and still persists today. The associated drastic consequences with respect to climate and geology forced us to adapt. Driven by necessity, the first pedestrians evolved in a kind of selection process based on the trial-and-error principle.

Eight million and more years ago, there were apes living in trees and moving exclusively on all fours. Skeletal finds prove that they were not anatomically equipped for walking upright. About 10 million years ago, some apes achieved such a high degree of dexterity in their longer front and shorter back limbs that they were able to change the way that they moved. Instead of walking on branches on all fours or leaping from branch to branch, they practiced the brachiating movement beneath the branches. The anatomical changes to front and back extremities as well as the pelvis that are necessary for this type of locomotion may have been the first step towards the subsequent biped posture.

Ardi is considered one of the first walkers. This 4.4 million year-old member of the species Ardipithicus ramidus was apparently able to walk on two legs, or at least that is what skeletal finds in Ethiopia point to. Reconstruction of the pelvis indicates that the woman, who weighed at least 51 kg (112 lbs.), was walking upright. However, her feet showed big toes that could be spread significantly, something that chimpanzees and gorillas do not have.

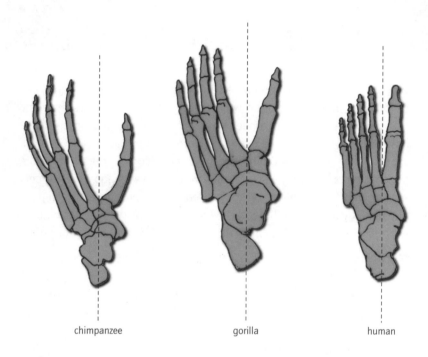

chimpanzee　　　　　gorilla　　　　　human

Fig. 2: Foot structure comparison between chimpanzees, gorillas, and humans

For the species Australopithecus that existed from approx. 4.4 million years ago until 2.3 million years ago, walking was pretty much a matter of course. Fossils verify that their bipedalism was fully developed, and their arm and leg fragments barely distinguishable from those of today's humans. The more than 3 million year-old skeletal finds of Lucy prove that she already traveled long distances on foot. Functional morphology studies prove that she was adapted to typical bipedal life on the ground based on the position of her big toes. The 3.6-million-year-old footprints are evidence that these prehistoric people were already able to roll their foot from heel to toe, and their ability to transfer weight and force is similar to our gait pattern.

Researchers consider these footprints irrefutable evidence of human bipedalism because the imprint depth of toes and heel, the resulting biomechanical motion sequence, and the energy efficiency already match that of the much younger Homo species. The research suggests that running was the energy-saving, yet versatile method of locomotion of humans as far back as 1.9 million years ago.

8 EVOLUTION OF BIPEDALISM

We can only speculate when and where exactly bipedalism became prevalent in humans. But there is proof that enormous evolutionary forces formed an upright-walking human from tree- and ground-dwelling apes. It is also undisputed that the morphological adaptation for upright bipedal locomotion necessitated considerable constructional changes to the skeleton. Without them, humans would not have been able to walk upright. Bipedalism required the most significant changes to the body structure that evolutionary biology is able to substantiate. Certain is that the upright gait made the use of the hands while walking superfluous, and simultaneously triggering a by all accounts momentous sociocultural evolution.

The evolution of bipedalism was as anatomically complex as it was seminal, in the truest sense of the word, adaptation for the evolution of humanity. The massive cranium moved backward to better balance on the now double-s-curve of the spine. The spine thereby formed the body axis that holds the head vertically over the hips while standing, and positions the trunk's center of gravity over the feet to maintain an equilibrium. The modified pelvis with wide, internally rotated iliac wings now offered suitable insertion areas for stronger gluteal and leg muscles. This changed the hip joint so that the legs with the elongated femoral neck came to stand vertically under the body, as a result enabling the extending and locking of the knee joint for effortless standing on feet, equipped with a strong big toe. But the enhanced, "tuned" hardware required the appropriate software and an adjustment to the control elements. This happened in the form of expanded and differentiated brain function and the vestibular organ in the ear that was specifically adapted to vertical space dimension.

9 FORM FOLLOWS FUNCTION

The innate, typical and compulsive human ability to walk on two legs is like a continuous rhythmic balancing act. It is an elaborately coordinated sequence of relinquishing and recovering equilibrium. Apes do not have that ability. The resulting possibilities of standing upright, using arms and hands independently, fundamentally separated us from our closest relatives. Long distances could be traveled with minimal energy expenditure while simultaneously carrying quarry. This development meant an even greater difference from our ancestors than the development of our cognitive, lingual, social, and cultural adaptations.

In many Olympic events, we come up short against the animal world in a direct comparison, but we are absolutely competitive in a combined event. We aren't the strongest and would not do well wrestling against an orangutan. We also aren't the fastest creatures on the planet and would be outrun by a number of mammals during the 100 m sprint. But our asset is versatility. An adult can hike 25 km without any real training. A sudden cloudburst can cause us to sprint 150 m to the next bus shelter, and then briskly walk another 1.5 km to the next pub. Climbing a tree, jumping across a creek, and swimming 200 m in a lake and even diving to a depth of 2 m, are also part of our repertoire of abilities, whereby swimming as we know was not an innate skill but one that had to be acquired with a technique.

For each of these skills, there is at least one animal that would beat us in a contest, but in all of these skills combined we are unbeatable. The ground-dwelling, upright human is also unbeatable when it comes to running long distances. Certain characteristics should be particularly emphasized here. The many sweat glands combined with less body hair proved extremely beneficial because heat would dissipate, preventing over-heating. Hunters took advantage of overheating and exhaustion and forced their four-legged prey to either rest or collapse. This factor accounted for the increased protein requirement precipitated by the major growth of brain and skull.

The incremental perfection of the hardware for bipedal locomotion and the associated modification of the software for motor abilities went hand in hand with the essential differentiation of the equilibrioception.

There are significant similarities between the species Homo ergaster that lived 1.9 million years ago, and modern day humans. The similarities with respect to height, weight, build, and proportions are primarily evidenced by their gait. Petrified footprints in Northern Kenya were analyzed. Those approx. 1.5 million year-old footprints showed without a doubt the hollow below the metatarsus that is typical to us, relatively short toes, and a large big toe that runs parallel to the other toes. The similarity to our customary gait could be verified based on the depth of the prints and the measurable stride length.

After the heel strike, the weight is shifted to the entire sole, and then rolls off via the ball of the foot to push off with the big toe. Moving upright on two legs thus seems indisputable and is natural as well as absolutely reasonable. Apart from any conjecture, there is even a clearly defined movement pattern.

10 LEARNING FROM NATURE

When we take a look around the animal kingdom and particularly the mammals related to us, it becomes clear that ground-dwelling animals have developed a form of movement that fits their lifestyle. Thus a cheetah moves differently than a crocodile, a chimpanzee or a horse, but they all use their feet in a species-specific manner and adapt their posture to the respective speed, i.e. the forces at work.

A horse, for instance, has four gaits. The horse is interesting because living in civilization like us means that it has to permanently wear shoes.

Horses are the only creatures that share our fate of having been born barefoot yet spend their lives in "shoes." They also share the problems created by footwear that is inappropriate for the species. When attaching a horseshoe, the natural wear of the keratin at the bottom of the hoof stops almost entirely, so that the horny box is gradually in an unnatural position relative to the ground. This is detrimental to the position of the limbs, the toes, and the shape of the hoof capsule, and as a result also affects the higher up parts of the extremities.

A horse's foundation is a healthy bare foot. The hoof provides sure footing on different terrain and facilitates effortless hoof wear during physiological loading of tendons, ligaments, and muscles. The ideal hoof construction, a combination of solid and elastic components, provides the perfect shock absorption. Moreover, the hoof supports the heart's transport of blood throughout the horse's body. After all, the horse feels the ground with its hoofs. Most of these abilities are impaired, or even rendered impossible by the use of permanent hoof protection. This applies, for instance, to the complete loss of shock absorption in the metal-shod hoof. The impairment of the hoof's natural abilities affects the horse's health and is a main cause of problems with the feet and musculoskeletal system.

The example of the horse clearly illustrates how muddled the situation is. Many people keep and love horses, sacrificing a lot of their precious free time to exercise the animals and spend money to rent stalls where their beloved four-legged friends are to live. These stalls are not very big, but have to be cleaned regularly and lined with shavings. The concept of modern horse-keeping does not seem logical when a flight and herd animal that requires a lot of space is locked in a narrow stall just to be taken for a walk or ridden in a circle a few times each day, instead of opening the stall door and turning the horses out together in a big pasture. There they can run, romp with their fellow species, and graze. Parallels to some of our fellow humans in urban centers are of course purely coincidental (See fig. 3, page 38).

When a horse begins to move, it first walks. It puts one hoof in front of the other and assumes the appropriate posture. When the horse accelerates, it moves into the next gait, the trot, and again adapts its outer shape and posture to the accelerating and soil reaction forces at work. As it begins to canter, it again changes automatically into the appropriate posture until it begins to gallop, and again assumes the appropriate posture.

"Nothing in biology makes sense
except in the light of evolution."

Theodosius Dobzhansky

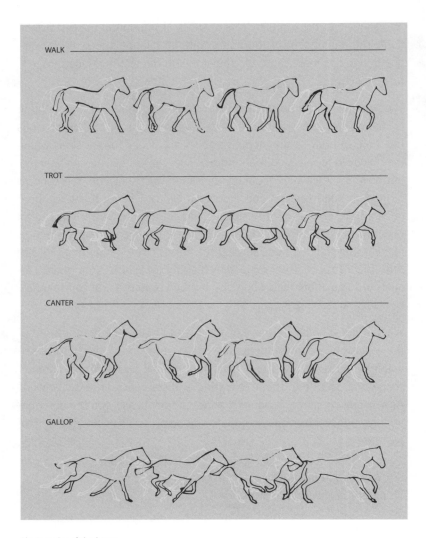

Fig. 3: Gaits of the horse

11 BIRDS FLY, FISH SWIM

Compared to a horse, the human has developed only three natural gaits for moving on the ground. Even today, we must choose from these three gaits for every task we have to complete in our daily lives or in sports. It doesn't matter if it is going to the bathroom in the morning, or running across the soccer pitch, or chasing after the bus.

Now it is important to understand how and why we move. From a physical point of view, movement is merely the interplay of gravity, ground reaction force, flexibility, and muscle action. They produce torque of the anatomical hinge joints within the skeletal system, meaning the joints. When there is sufficient torque, the bones move and trigger a movement.

Human locomotion is essentially generating and controlling torque. Human performance and injuries are linked to the ability to generate and control torque in the joints. Walking, running, and sprinting are visually different adaptations to different speeds and the resulting greater gravitational and soil reaction forces.

While walking, the forces that affect our locomotor system are relatively minor. When switching to the next-faster gait, running, the load doubles and triples, and finally increases to up to ten times the bodyweight while sprinting. Failure of the joint positions adjusting to the respective forces would inevitably lead to overloading and injury.

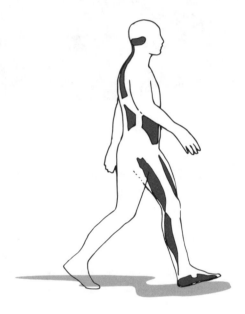

Fig. 4: Walking

The first gait, walking, involves pendular leg-movement. We shift our weight from one leg to the other. Since one foot always has contact with the ground, only our basic bodyweight affects our structure and the contact with the ground is relatively long. The soil contact time is relevant because it delineates the period of time that the foot makes contact with the ground. The longer the soil contact time, meaning the amount of time the foot and the superior structures have available to handle the occurring load and adjust to it, the easier it is. While walking, we have lots of time under a minor load. Walking is therefore the easiest form of locomotion.

The effectiveness of an upright gait is regularly challenged in casual conversation, and even some "experts" consider bipedalism an evolutionary error or believe to have recognized the natural form of movement in the completely abnormal forefoot strike.

If we divide walking into so-called *cycles*, we have one swinging leg and one standing leg for every cycle. In doing so, one leg acts as the swinging leg and does not make contact with the ground, but instead swings forward. The other leg is the standing or supporting leg that maintains contact with the ground. This reverses during the next cycle.

While walking, the leg swings forward from the hip joint and gently plants the heel in front of the body's center of gravity.

The foot must be flexed (dorsal flexion) as the leg swings forward, otherwise it would drag on the ground. When the heel strikes, the point where it makes contact with the ground becomes a leverage point for a lever, or more simply put a *seesaw*. It is a seesaw because the diagonally downward acting soil contact force and gravity cause the foot to fold forward without wasting any energy.

This so-called *calcaneus seesaw* leads to increased tension in the calf caused by the kinetic chain of the myofascial tissue. It is essentially the pretension that builds up with the flexing of the foot and now unloads due to the involved connective tissue's elasticity. Like a lever with the ankle acting as the fulcrum, the shin, knee, thigh, and subsequently the hip are flung forward. This inverted pendulum represents the basic principle of vibration theory, and the kinetic levers make the human gait so efficient.

PLEASE NOTE

Gravity, soil reaction force, elasticity, and muscle reaction create torque in the anatomical hinge joints of the skeletal system, meaning in the joints. If the torque is great enough, the bones move, triggering motion.

Human locomotion is essentially generating and controlling torque. Human performance and injuries are linked to the ability to generate and control torque in the joints.

12 THE ACTIVE GAIT

To take a step forward, the human has to shift his center of gravity forward and transmit force. This requires firm contact with the ground, comparable to a sprinter who uses a starting block to transmit the strength of his legs to the ground via the active structures. The last link in this kinetic chain is the big toe, which, due to his higher bone density, greater mobility, and strong muscles, is perfectly equipped for the job.

The big toe with help from his smaller colleagues transfers the leg's strength to the ground. With every step he makes sure that the body's forward tilt generates propulsion. Walking is nothing other than the forward shifting of bodyweight from one leg to the other. But in order for forward movement to occur, momentum must be generated from the ground to create propulsion.

But first the heel makes gentle contact with the ground in front of the center of gravity, and the foot is then flexed. This pretension (dorsal flexion) is important to subsequently be able to efficiently push off in the opposite direction, similar to bending the knees before jumping. Now that the center of gravity has moved farther forward, the foot is lowered slightly to the outside (supination) in the direction of the little toe. The body now stands over the foot so that the entire foot is needed on the ground.

The big toe takes the lead, and wants to reestablish contact with the ground, tilting the foot to the inside (pronation). The big toe immediately takes over and with his strength prevents excessive pronation. The body moves farther forward and the toe maintains contact, the metatarsophalangeal joint of the big toe hinges down and finally actively pushes, but due to the pretension in the plantar fascia, also develops a kind of elastic recoil that is relatively small but "nice to have," making the progressive motion more efficient.

If you take the time to sit in an outdoor café and watch the pedestrians without contemplating their fashion-sense or secondary sexual characteristics, you will notice that the human gait often has little to do with the gait of the Homo sapiens, but rather more that of the chimpanzee even though they rarely and inefficiently move on two legs. Chimpanzees don't move very economically on two legs because their hips, knees, and ankles do not possess the critical specifications. They did not receive these over the course of evolution. A chimpanzee therefore walks rather clumsily and very obviously shifts his weight from side to side. Chimpanzees also switch to bipedalism only when they want to impress and not just get from A to B.

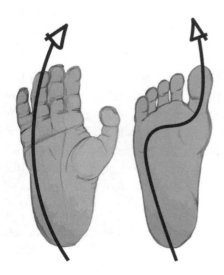

Fig. 5: Foot comparison, chimpanzee and human

Modern humans have forgotten how to walk and their shoes are to blame. Next to the aforementioned heel lift that causes us to pitch forward, destroying our structural stability, and forcing the knees, hips, and lumbar spine to compensate, shoes have another incomprehensible feature: the pointed and raised toe box.

This places the big toe in a kind of stand-by mode for hours each day causing its autonomous muscle nourishment to adapt. When active use of the toes is no longer possible, the toes are raised and the body forgoes its toe function and relies only on the middle and hind foot to carry the bodyweight.

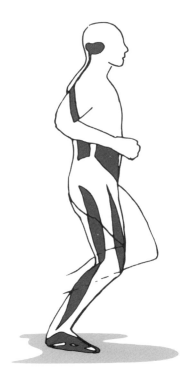

Fig. 6: Running

While running, the forces at work change, along with the soil contact time. Running is nothing other than jumping from one leg to the other while using the elastic properties of Achilles tendon and plantar fascia. Under certain conditions, this is very economical. Due to the acceleration, the soil reaction force has doubled or even tripled while the soil contact time has been halved. This results in increased complexity, meaning a greater load must be processed in less time, requiring more highly developed skill than just walking.

PLEASE NOTE:

Locomotion can be seen as "controllable" instability with phases of stability and instability. The shorter the stability phase, the greater the necessary neuromuscular control.

Walking (60% soil contact during a cycle)

Running (40% soil contact during a cycle)

Here it is surprising that in spite of the high and higher load during the switch from the first gait walking to the second gait running, comparatively fewer muscles are recruited, and correspondingly less muscle strength is required. This in turn implies a considerably lower likelihood of overloading or injury.

When changing gaits, the human being also changes his shape and the changed posture results from a changed joint position, a different movement sequence of the limbs, leading to modulation in the myofascial tissues, which offset the increased muscular effort with increased elasticity.

When sprinting, the parameters change again due to the high tempo. The load increases to up to ten times the bodyweight, and the amount of time the foot is on the ground has been shortened quite a bit. That is also why sprinting is the most complex gait and the supreme discipline we rarely choose for a reason, and one I can sustain for only a very short amount of time.

In summary, there is a typical load for every type of locomotion as well as a corresponding posture we must assume to be able to move efficiently and injury-free.

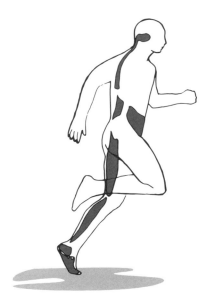

Fig. 7: Human sprint

13 SIXTH SENSE – PROPRIOCEPTION

Luckily we don't have to worry about that because our body controls these processes and in doing so relies on the information provided by the sensory organs and receptors.

Just like in those first driving lessons, here, too, the question arises with respect to our locomotion of when should we shift into what gear to avoid crossing the rpm redline? We would need a tachometer to decide when to shift based on the rotational frequency. Being aware of body position and movement in space is a critical factor for a good strike and injury-free movement.

These mechanoreceptors are sensitive end organs that respond to the status and changes of the locomotor system and supporting structures, but also affect the other receptors that signal the status and status changes of the own body. A large portion of these can be found in the sole of the foot, which is completely logical since our feet provide the only contact we have with the ground.

The sensory contact with the ground is also the quickest link to transmitting information regarding the condition, temperature, and structure of the ground we move on. Surface irregularities that require active adjustments in the ankle, knee, or hip are immediately processed reflexively by the central nervous system instead of being transferred to the, by comparison, relatively sluggish visual conduit.

Every running stride generates extreme stress and strain. If those forces aren't absorbed, it can lead to injuries to the musculoskeletal system because the forces occur faster than the muscles can react. Study results show that the maximum effect occurs within 10-30 milliseconds. But muscles need at least 40 milliseconds to contract. Here intensive training of the thigh musculature, which is always promoted as the solution, plays a minor part in protecting the knee from the stress while jogging.

Our body relies on our feet. It is similar to modern cars that permanently resort to their robot assistance system for drive train information. Feelers and sensors collect data so they can intervene in a borderline situation. Electronic stability programs and anti-lock braking systems are standard equipment and can be turned off with the push of a button whenever the experienced driver wants to deliberately test the limits. But for most drivers, the assistants are permanently switched on and do their job reliably and imperceptibly. They do so imperceptibly at 30 mph on a dry road, or violently intervene at 110 mph while hydroplaning during a lane change.

Our feet fight on the frontlines against any surface we move on and absorb any kind of stress and strain with their longitudinal and transverse arch. More specifically, it is less like a battle and more like a constant arranging by activating muscles and fascial structures, the plantar fascia and the Achilles tendon. This does not happen actively but unconsciously. Consciously controlling each of these compensating motions would downright overwhelm us. That is the job of the sole of the foot.

14 PLASTIC FOAM WONDERLAND

Only in the past 50 years, have we been continuously packing new and better constructed layers of plastic foam equipped with dubious functional components under the soles of our feet. In the firm belief that our feet need cushioning and stability provided by shoes, we close our eyes to the fact that plastic foam et al. only keep our feet from doing their evolutionarily hereditary job.

Hi-tech plastic foam only cushion the sensation and flow of information, but not the force effect. These layers of trash make an efficient force transmission to the ground impossible. It is like trying to bounce a basketball on a gym mat. A healthy foot brings with it all the technology that we need. The cushioning and wealth of functions propagated by the sporting goods industry is promoted as the ultimate remedy, which probably applies more to the manufacturers than the people.

Moreover, the footbed and support elements make our feet dumb and lazy because feet need everything but a bed. Any existing abilities diminish day by day until people can no longer walk or run without shoes and ankle support.

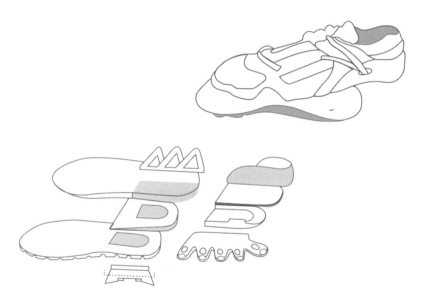

Fig. 8: "Hi-tech" that is actually "low-tech" for the feet

15 JOGGING & THE ACHILLES HEEL

When this data is missing in a complex system like our body that depends on sufficient information and feedback to be able to move, it creates problems. One of them is jogging.

In literature, the term *jogging* first appeared in the book with the same title. Before that there was no jogging and people simply ran. Jogging is the brainchild of the University of Oregon athletic coach Bill Bowerman, who published the book titled *Jogging* in 1964. The power of the written word, backed by nice photographs and illustrations, motivated people to replace their formerly natural running style with a hybrid form of walking and running, and henceforth they went jogging. An important characteristic of jogging that stood out was the happy roll over. The foot was supposed to make contact leading with the heel and then roll over onto the toes. Its logic is similar to that of today's Nordic walking, another successful attempt at selling people on an unnatural way of moving and the corresponding products under the guise of health promotion. The Nordic walking trend made hiking poles the popular accessory of courageously tromping hordes in our parks.

Thus jogging is not an innate ability but, at a closer look, not only counterproductive for the purpose of locomotion, but also a fatal strain on our bodies.

The heel strike in front of the body's center of gravity, no matter how gentle or skillful, will slow the body down and bring it to a complete standstill. The principle of the heel striking in front of the body's center of gravity is otherwise only known in skiing or sledding in order to decelerate or stop. To continue to move this neutral point must be overcome with lots of muscular effort. This effort doesn't just make jogging strenuous but is an inappropriate strain and overload. Most of the time the average jogger will complain of regular knee or hip pain, back problems, or shoulder pain. Justifiably, since we know that enormous forces equivalent to approximately three times our bodyweight come to bear when jumping from one leg to the other.

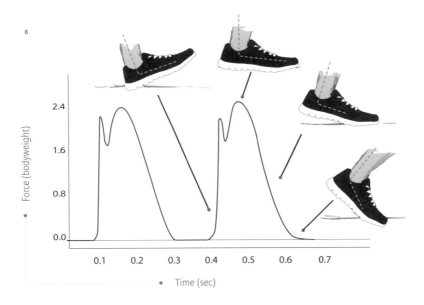

Fig. 9: Amount of force on the foot – barefoot – with athletic shoes – correct gait

The amount of force during the heel strike with a nearly straight leg is so great that it practically drives into the entire structure. This means regular overloading of the muscles and participating joints, from the heel bone, to the Achilles tendon, ankle, shin, knee, patellar tendon, all the way to the hip (SIJ), lumbar spine, and higher up to the chest and shoulder-girdle, and the neck muscles that have to support the massive skull in an unnatural forward-leaning posture.

To further clarify the problem with jogging, let's imagine that it's raining and you don't feel like running in the rain. But you are motivated and really want to run. So instead of going out in the rain, you lie down on your living room floor and raise your legs with the soles of the feet facing the ceiling. Assuming you weigh 154 lb. and take an average 100 strides per minute, you now ask someone with a 463 lb. sledgehammer to alternate striking each heel 50 times. As strange as that might sound, aside from the cardiovascular activity, that is what a round of jogging does to your body.

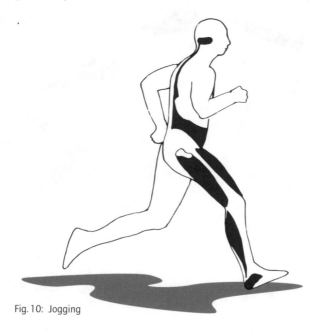

Fig. 10: Jogging

When you look at the average jogger in the wild, in parks and on river trails, next to the colorful tights and compression socks, the headlamp, and the GPS-equipped heart rate monitors, you can see by the expression on his face that he isn't having much fun.

Bowerman had created a system with his book that back then was only marginally successful. In those days, the first jogger suffered from heel pain because there weren't any tennis shoes with heel cushions. So after Bowerman had created a problem, his next step was to offer a solution. Using his wife's old waffle iron, he developed a shoe sole with a plastic foam heel in his basement, the first jogging shoe, then had a university student design a logo and named the company after the Greek goddess of victory, Nike. The company still sells athletic shoes that make jogging as comfortable as possible for your heels.

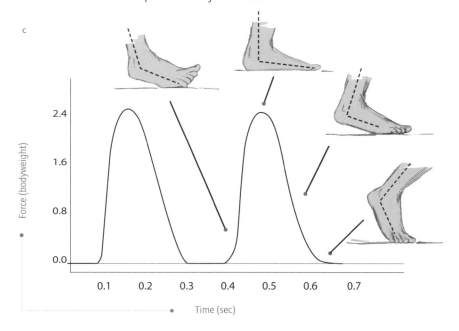

Fig. 11: Amount of force on the foot – correct gait

Interesting in this context are the similarities to American football. In the NFL, the North American professional league, concussions are as common as bruises in soccer. Studies have shown that an above-average number of players suffer from neuropsychological disorders. While the helmets they wear protect their skulls from injury, they can prevent neither concussion nor buffer the effects of massive collision forces on the cervical spine. The long-term effects are dramatic and studies show a significantly higher risk of severe neurological disorders like Alzheimer's, Parkinson's, or brain tumors.

16 HARDWARE – SOFTWARE

You have forgotten how to run, but a copy of the lost software is still on your hard drive.

Take a simple test at your own risk. Stand upright and jump up with both feet. Do it several times in a row like jumping rope, just without the rope. Now pay attention to how you land and which part of the foot you land on.

Did you land on your forefoot? Try and see what it feels like to land on your heels. You can wear shoes if you like.

The fact is, no one would voluntarily land on the heels. Even with athletic shoes it doesn't feel good. So why do we do it?

We are born runners but the husbandry conditions have worsened over time. A free-range system on the ground has turned into a cage system. Chairs and shoes force us into a relieving posture, and the hardware, our hunter-gatherer body, suffers under the flawed operating system. The result is conflict and incompatibility.

Running and jogging, or other forms of exercise are strongly discouraged in this condition because you will get hurt. Forget running! You probably won't even be able to stand anymore.

17 BACK TO THE START – FACTORY SETTING

Regardless of how good and effective the hardware is, what matters for performance is the software. You are familiar with this from your smart phone or PC that always downloads new updates. Unfortunately we installed inferior software, a faulty operating system, which leads to the hardware-software incompatibility.

A visit to the zoo illustrates this problem quite well. The big cat in the obviously too-small cage continuously paces back and forth on its beaten path with empty eyes and a dull coat. The cage most likely even meets the minimum requirements for keeping big cats in zoos, but neither the cage nor the cat look like it. I would love to open the cage door and tell the cat: "Run, Kitty, run!" and watch it disappear in the nearby forest. But in reality, big cats are genetically still big cats, and it is only their adaption to their housing conditions which has "impaired" them to a degree that they would most likely starve or wait to die from injuries within a few days. And this is simply all because they have forgotten how to be a big cat.

That or similar is how it is with us modern humans. The zoo-human in overpopulated urban centers with too little living space does not have a species-appropriate diet, is depressed, unable to reproduce, and has forgotten how to stand, walk, and run.

These innate abilities must be rekindled step-by-step following the natural movement hierarchy, first standing, then walking, and finally running. Like all natural systems, human locomotion builds on simple patterns that become increasingly more complex. Just like a child that first belly-crawls, then crawls on all fours, stands, walks, and runs.

If you have worn shoes throughout your life, your feet are too weak. That's why we will do what they do with a big cat that is first placed in a reintroduction program in order for it to be able to gradually relearn all abilities.

18 MOVEMENT MILESTONES

All of us have learned to move at some point. And we have done so without taking a class, reading a manual, or watching a YouTube video tutorial.

Infants have an innate desire to move that lends them the will and strength to roll from the unpopular supine position over onto their stomach. Once they have rolled over on their stomach, the entertainment doesn't just consist of looking at the ceiling or the colorful mobile. Once on the stomach, the massive head must be lifted and stabilized. It's a highly intense workout that develops the abilities for subsequent actions.

In a prone position, the field of vision has expanded and many interesting things can now be discovered. These beg to be looked at and examined more closely. That means propulsion must be generated somehow. Like seals, human babies activate their lower and upper extremities to push themselves across the room on their bellies so they can reach electrical outlets, cabinets, or shoes.

Once that has been accomplished, we want more and try to lift the still relatively heavy upper body by pushing up onto our forearms. Then we sit up at some point and learn for the first time what balance is. Holding the upper body upright alone is a highly complex process.

Once we have mastered sitting up, we begin to crawl to more closely examine the new visual impressions. This level of mobility often exceeds the resilience of the parental range of motion. If the offspring was here just moments ago, it is now someplace completely different.

When crawling is slow to develop, the parents in particular tend to get impatient. After all, we did not pass down our excellent fashion sense to the next generation for nothing and have endowed little Nicholas with a pair of Nike Air Max and a matching baseball cap at birth. On Saturday, during the firmly established outing to the city, the pedestrian zone becomes a runway and Junior has to come along. Unfortunately, he is completely uninterested and doesn't care about his parents' fashion sense either.

His caring parents take him in the middle and little Nicholas, who would rather crawl, is dragged through the pedestrian zone. Crawling trains coordination between the two halves of the body and little Nicholas was not allowed to practice it sufficiently. This is something that will become a factor during the next developmental step when the first large ball flies towards Nicholas. Once we stand, the first major movement milestone has been mastered.

Standing is one of the three major movement skills. What does standing have to do with movement? As bipedal beings, we are in a constant state of precarious equilibrium and must find and maintain our balance via unconsciously controlled muscular effort. For this process, we rely on as much information as possible about the ground beneath our feet.

We have all learned to stand, usually barefoot and in accordance to our individual stage of development, whether after 7 or 15 months. Once we have mastered keeping our balance, we become overconfident, relinquishing and regaining our newly acquired balance by putting one foot in front of the other. This is called walking. Once we have mastered this, we move faster and begin to run until we run fast, i.e. sprint.

So there is a specific sequence to learning to move. As is generally valid in training theory, we learn to move from easy to difficult, from simple to complex. This hierarchy of movement skills is not an option but rather an important sequence that builds on itself to optimally develop the locomotor system and avoid errors or limitations in the hardware-software connection.

This means we must first stand, then walk, and finally run to avoid injuries and prevent overloading, regardless of whether the colorful photos and snappy slogans of the sporting goods industry and the co-opted trade press want to get us to a half or full marathon within ten weeks.

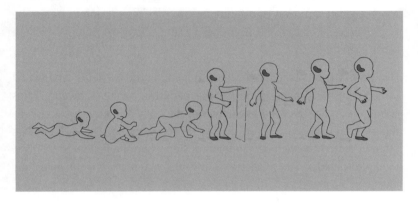

Fig. 12: Movement milestones in child development: from crawling to standing to walking

19 WE HAVE FORGOTTEN HOW TO STAND

Most people are no longer able to stand. Our bipedalism has many advantages but the flipside of the coin is that in order to master balance, we have to put in a lot of effort. Heels, and I am not talking about women's 3-inch heels, sabotage this ability to such a degree that we have to make a huge effort to stand upright.

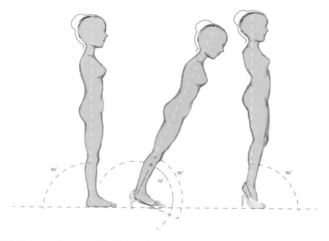

Fig. 13: Unnatural stance with high heels

Today, everyone without exception wears shoes with some kind of heel. Some now feel like this doesn't apply to them or they feel like they are being treated unfairly. "I only wear flats," is what I hear time and time again. The ladies then point to their ballerina slippers that often have a raised heel, and upon closer inspection, have little to do with the shape of our feet. It looks much more like a bitter battle against the ballerina that almost causes the ballerina to burst. Regardless of how high the heel is, we refer to a *heel lift*, meaning the heel is higher than the forefoot.

This now slanted base initially throws us off balance. It has probably been a few weeks since you built a tower with blocks, but if you were to build one today, you would probably do so on a level surface and not place a wedge beneath it.

In humans, the heel destroys our hard-fought equilibrium and causes the body to be off-balance.

The raised heel, even if it lifts the heel only half an inch, actually causes us to pitch forward. To avoid falling forward, we have to adjust. The urgently needed joint alignment to counter gravity results in a compensatory postural adjustment.

We compensate for the altered supporting surface with compensatory movements of the knees, hips, and spine, destroying the body's once so effective alignment. Joints are no longer lined up, muscle chains and fascial structures can no longer efficiently transfer force or utilize it via their elastic properties. The result is the phenomenon known in material science as tension that leads to overloading, injury, and ultimately pain.

What other explanation is there for pain caused by a relatively simple activity like standing? A heel's right to exist can be derived from its equestrian origins and the use of stirrups, but for ground-dwelling apes it is strictly an impediment and is pointless.

20 STABILITY

Humans love *stability*. Stability is a key factor in our existence on this planet because with only two legs, we have to permanently balance our upright body.

We are particularly aware of this fact after having a few alcoholic drinks, when we gradually lose our hard-earned stability and begin to sway. Within only a few hours, the ways in which we made it from a crawling infant to an upright walking adult are forgotten and we are not just figuratively back to moving on all fours. The movement milestones are lost.

The position of a focal point with regard to the support surface is critical to the body's vertical stability. A body can only stand on its support surface if the plumb line meets it, meaning when the support surface is below the center of mass. If that is not the case, the body will tip over.

PLEASE NOTE:

Center of gravity

The body's center of gravity is the point at which the body's total weight is in effect. The bodyweight acts from the center of gravity vertically downward along a line (the bodyweight line of action).

Every part of the human body has a center of gravity.

During a certain posture or movement, the body acts like the total weight of all its parts is concentrated on one single point. That point is the general center of gravity or general center of mass.

Our feet form our body's support surface. To keep us from falling over, we must continuously balance our upright posture. This balancing activity is the job of the sole of the foot.

When we move, we first shift our center of gravity across the support surface, the soles of our feet, and our body then begins to fall over.

Once our body falls, it desperately wants to check that movement with a counter-movement to regain stability.

Thus even the upright stance requires continuous movement. It brings back childhood memories of playing with game pieces that didn't want to stand up.

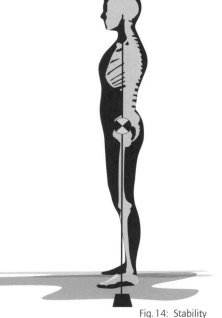

Fig. 14: Stability

The human body as a two-legged body can perform many more movements than the game pieces and even quadrupeds. Good examples of our body's abilities are gymnasts and acrobats. When a gymnast concludes his floor routine with a double flip and sticks the landing, he isn't wearing a cushioning plastic foam wedge under his feet. He relies on the abilities of his feet and the soles. He depends on the soles of his feet to provide the necessary stability during every landing or on the balance beam. Gymnasts don't wear shoes because those would impede efficient movement and the gathering of takeoff power.

Thus every single movement must be regulated by the sole of the foot so we don't fall over, and that is the case whether I am sweating in a Zumba class, doing deadlifts, or just going from machine to machine according to my workout plan.

That means the foot isn't just for walking. Sole of the foot impairment can explain many medical conditions and disorders above the ankles.

PLEASE NOTE:

Definition of stability

A body is considered stable when the action line of its body-weight is within the area of its base of support.

21 THE THREE PILLARS

Next to the video analysis on the treadmill that gives us information about our running technique and gait, the *pressure measurement plate* is a very important tool for analyzing the position and function of the foot. The pressure measurement plate measures the pressure of the foot or rather the sole transfers to the ground, meaning the amount of force the foot exerts on its support surface. The different pressure areas are displayed in different colors, whereby blue indicates low pressure, green-yellow indicates higher pressure, and red indicates very high pressure.

The standard pressure image of a normal person when he takes off his shoes and stands on the plate will show high pressure on the ball of the foot and relatively high pressure on the heel. The big toes will barely, or not at all, produce a pressure point. Even after being asked and attempting to press the big toes into the ground, pressure increases very little.

Due to its outstanding abilities with respect to strength and mobility as compared to the smaller toes, the big toe is the most important link in the kinematic chain of the lower extremities. However, this is not just in terms of progressive movement. While standing, everything relies on the big toe, and thus the ability to press the big toe into the ground is a prerequisite for stability while standing.

The ball of the foot is the second pillar and together with the third pillar, the heel, they form the foundation of the arch and greatly contribute to the correct foot alignment. In order to optimally contribute bodyweight, ensure the function of the arch, and transfer the force to the ground, a healthy foot must have these three Pillars: the big toe, the ball of the foot, and the heel. Similar to a tripod, we too, don't just stand on two feet; rather our feet rest on three pillars. Two pillars aren't steady enough and even four table legs can wobble on an uneven surface.

That is impossible with three legs, and thus our feet also adhere to this principle. Sadly, we are barely able to build all three pillars anymore, and as a result the sole of the foot is also overloaded. When our bodyweight rests on only two pillars, most often the ball of the foot and the heel, our stance is rather unstable. When the big toe isn't sufficiently activated, it is unable to adequately deploy its critical function and strength. The result is pressure pain, particularly in the forefoot and the sensitive metatarsal bones. Even while just standing, the big toe is painfully missed.

PLEASE NOTE:

Definition of instability

A body is considered unstable when the action line of its bodyweight is outside the area of its support base.

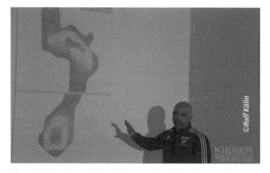

Fig. 15: The three pillars, big toe, ball of the foot, and heel bone

22 IF YOU WANT TO WALK YOU HAVE TO BE ABLE TO STAND

When working with thousands of active and aspiring joggers, the *treadmill analysis* is the first step to determining the status quo. Here we differentiate three types.

22.1 THE AVERAGE JOGGER

You generally see him on river promenades, on the lakeshore, or along forest trails. The latter primarily for damping-purposes because the soft forest floor is easy on the joints. While faith may move mountains, it does not protect us from the effects of gravity. The generally brief jogging experience begins in the spring, equipped with tights, a headlamp, hydration belt, GPS heart monitor, compression socks, and of course the latest model from the plastic foam wonderland. The desire for forward propulsion is abruptly interrupted by the heel strike against the ground. This dead point must now be overcome with lots of effort and muscle strength, only to create complete stoppage again.

The load peak in a structure, not intended for this purpose, is the cause for many injuries like shin splints, jogger knee, or irritated meniscus.

Next to the heel strike which is only possible with the appropriately cushioned footwear – try it: jump barefoot onto your heels! – your posture matters. Long strides with nearly straight legs, bending at the hip, head forward, and lots of arm action.

22.2 THE BAREFOOT ENTHUSIAST

Barefoot running has arrived in health magazines and has been around for some time on the running scene, unleashed by Christopher McDougall's bestseller *Born to Run*. Forefoot running learned on YouTube or in a quick barefoot running class usually leads to massive problems with the Achilles tendon and metatarsal bones.

The unfamiliar stress and strain generated by several hundred jumps from one leg to the other, without the appropriate relaxation and the gentle contact of the heel with the ground, doesn't just clench the calf muscles but causes the already preloaded Achilles tendon to bow out with a bang.

But he won't be deterred. He has understood that barefoot is good, and the barefoot running shoes have already been ordered.

22.3 THE RELAXED UPRIGHT BAREFOOT RUNNER

The evolution of the average jogger to barefoot enthusiast is complete. Upright body, the foot strikes below and slightly behind the body's center of gravity. As with a foot-bike, the foot strike creates constant propulsion and accelerates the body's forward movement, receiving the momentum in an efficient manner.

23 NORMAL, BUT NOT NATURAL

There are many things in this world that don't make sense, and sometimes the search for meaning isn't appropriate. But what has driven the shoe industry to manufacture clothing for our feet, something that is not at all in line with the anatomy of our feet, is a mystery. When you look down at yourself, you will either see shoes that have nothing in common with your feet's anatomy, or you will see feet that are shaped like their shoes.

And it's so simple. Human feet are wide in the front and narrow in the back. The forefoot with the ball of the foot and the toes is wider than the bony, slightly cushioned heel bone. Under pressure, the five toes spread like a fan and the big toe facilitates stability on the inside of the foot and the transfer of force from the leg to the ground. Two thirds of all leg muscles come together in the big toe, and the bone is thicker and denser than those of the smaller toes. But modern footwear permanently forces the big toe from its hereditary position towards the smaller toes or rather over or under them, where it withers in insignificance. Furthermore, an upward-sloped sole profile causes it to hang motionless in the toe of the shoe without contact with the ground. Even if it still had any strength, it wouldn't have a chance against the firm soles of most shoes.

The shelves at sporting goods stores are filled with lots of creations by the design and research departments of large corporations. Consumers are no longer able to handle the number of models, concepts and absolutely necessary functions alone. The fear of buying the wrong shoe based on esthetic characteristics is much too great. The plastic foam wonderland tempts the target group of overweight joggers, sick overpronators, and minimalists driven by the heart monitor with more cushioning, more support and better performance.

The truth is, neither boost, air, gel, nor spring-loaded soles can make those destructive momenta caused by jumping from one heel to the other disappear. The only thing these layers of trash do is dull the sensation of the sole, i.e. reduce the pain of the heel strikes. Damaged feet without sufficient sensation, without the necessary ankle mobility, and without full function of the big toe, lead to strange motion sequences. Motivated by pure greed for profit, clever marketing constantly presents us with new models made with better and more sophisticated technology which still don't change the high percentage of injured runners (soccer players). This arms race might make some people feel like they've done all that they can. But the result remains unsatisfactory.

Even in other human forms of movement, lots of effort and good materials don't necessarily mean success. When there is too much cushioning and a lack of sensation, many things fall by the wayside. As much protection as possible for as much sensation as possible doesn't just make procreation, but also propulsion of adventure.

Runners, and particularly performance-oriented runners, like to believe in the promises of the industry to make up for their lack of physical prerequisites with technical ones, even it they are minimally helpful. The sporting goods industry has been preaching this for too long and has validated this dogma with the performances of their masterful mercenaries among the world's elite.

24 WHERE THE SHOE PINCHES

But shoes weren't always bad for us. In fact, in the beginning they made a lot of sense and served to protect the sensitive sole of the foot from injury and weather conditions like extreme cold and heat.

If we go on the assumption that the cradle of civilization lies in East Africa, the species Homo has explored the entire planet from there on foot.

But the first footwear, developed about 40,000 years ago, clearly shows that next to its function, the shoe design was primarily based on the shape of the foot.

Today it is unfortunately the opposite, and the foot conforms to the shape of the shoe.

Remember how much your children enjoyed putting on shoes for the first time? There was lots of crying because the shoes pinched.

When you try on shoes, you initially feel like the shoes pinch, but after some encouragement from the salesclerk and the familiar phenomenon that the shoes merely have to be broken in, you buy them anyway. But why do we buy shoes that don't fit or take time to get comfortable? Because that's how it is and always has been, as well as there being a lack of alternatives.

One of the most successful shoe models of recent years is the *Nike Free*. It was a great shoe that took advantage of the barefoot trend and promised freedom for the feet. But upon closer examination, this freedom is deceptive because the last, meaning the shape of the sole, is basically the same as your off-the-shelf jogging shoe. However, it was the structure of the sole that was something special. Notches divided the sole into blocks and thereby allowed an exceptional amount of flexibility, making it possible to completely roll up the shoe and pull the toes up all the way to the ankle. But here is the question: when was the last time you rolled up your foot and where is the benefit when this movement is incompatible with the sole itself?

In addition, there is still a built-in heel lift, meaning the heel is higher than the forefoot, which results in the familiar loss of stability, i.e. we actually fall forward and have to use lots of effort to compensate.

And then there was the MBT shoe, an extremely ugly specimen with a massive, semi-circular convex sole, that was sold as a cure for back pain, propagating the return to the natural roll-off the way the Massai practice it. Hence the name MBT, short for Massai Barefoot Technology. The insanity behind this name must have been extensive because when you do a Google search of Massai, you notice that none of the Massai in the photos wears MBTs.

And they also don't produce them or have any involvement with this product. They were simply used to link a healthy, natural way of moving to this grotesque spawn of the shoe industry.

But I have received the occasional feedback that the effect is positive and back pain seemed to have gone away. A similar shoe, Reebok's *Easy Tone*, even promised a tight behind, but was discontinued after a lawsuit by a dissatisfied customer whose backside apparently didn't respond to Easy Tone.

But what the MBT did accomplish was remarkable. The sole construction produced such a diffuse muscle tone, a. o. in the hip-flexor muscles and around the spine and caused the pain receptors in the connective tissue to get so overloaded, that the back pain disappeared. A slap in the face would have produced a similar result, but have been harder to sell. The stress the MBT produced was so great that it obscured any pain, and could be attributed to the fact that people love stability and therefore like to stand on firm ground. When the ground moves, it is a signal to quickly return to the cave and wait until the earthquake is over instead of carrying it with us.

I briefly want to talk about high heels, but only briefly because they are not the problem. High heels are not comfortable, even if their passionate wearers stubbornly deny this fact, and compared to all the other types of shoes are actually worn quite rarely. Fortunately high heels are so inherently uncomfortable that the amount of time the foot can tolerate them is predictable. Much worse are tennis shoes, leather shoes for the office, and ballerina flats, because all of them ignore and disregard the foot's anatomy in the most contemptible way.

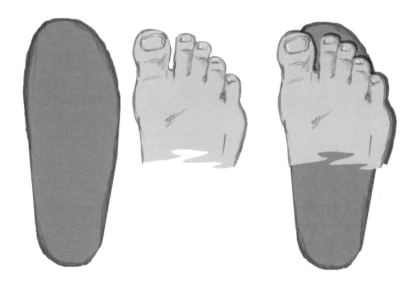

Fig. 16: The fit of conventional shoes: what's wrong with this fit?

25 FROM HEAD TO TOE

The body is a complete work of art, and muscles initiate every one of our body's movements. Our muscles don't just facilitate our progressive movement but also vital functions such as the heartbeat and respiration.

To be able to move, our body's muscles must shorten and relax. This shortening or relaxing is transferred to the adjacent bone, which then moves the joint and transfers the movement from there to the next muscle. This process is repeated until the muscle's effort produces the intended effect somewhere outside the body.

It is the responsibility of the *fasciaes* to transfer muscle force because they envelop every muscle and every organ like a thin membrane, and form tendons, ligaments, and joint capsules.

This connective tissue consists of collagen fibers, and like all of the body's structures it is very efficient, but also very adaptable. This adaptability is both a blessing and a curse. For many hours each day several days a week, our predominantly seated posture primarily places our active structures in a position that is inconsistent with our upright locomotion. Standing upright gets increasingly difficult and muscles, tendons, and ligaments shorten more and more. This shortening or muscle tension has a proven performance-decreasing effect and the high number of receptors in the connective tissue signal pain.

This in turn, leads to a lack of efficiency and restricted mobility, meaning the joints are no longer able to move through their complete range of motion, and muscle use is limited.

Regardless of which action we perform with the strength of our muscles, the purpose will always lie outside the body. So there is always an overriding function or result behind every muscle action like, for instance, standing up, lifting, pulling up, pushing away, bending, extending. We generally have the use of our limbs, our upper and lower extremities, to transfer this muscle power. In addition to their balancing function, legs and feet in particular are constantly used to transfer and discharge forces.

When these forces don't completely transfer, due to the above mentioned limitation, they must somehow be processed and used in situ. This unforeseen force effect must then be handled for a corresponding accommodation to take place.

26 PUNISHMENT COMES HARD ON THE HEELS

A body is only as strong as its foundation. As any architect can confirm, it makes sense, contrary to popular opinion, that our core, our trunk, and especially our deep muscles are the critical factor for our performance capacity to build our house from the bottom up. Let's begin with the foundation before we build the upper floor and walls.

Next to the function of the big toe and the big toe flexor, the rest of the 33 muscles are so atrophied or at least greatly restricted, that efficient movement is difficult. In addition to a sufficiently exercised musculature, efficient movement is based on fascial structures, the connective tissue that envelops and connects all of our muscles and joints and permeates the entire body from the big toe to the hairline. Fascia research promoted by Dr. Robert Schleip, is based on findings that were gained from the ground up, i.e. the fascia of the foot and calf. Specifically the plantar and Achilles aponeurosis were examined via ultrasound.

The function of the plantar fascia can be thought of as a shock absorber. The plantar fascia, which runs the length of the bottom of the foot, makes sure that when the foot is loaded, pressure and impact are not transferred unchecked to the muscles and nerves of the foot. When wearing modern shoes, cushioning and pronation support greatly relieve pressure on the plantar fascia, shortening it as a result. The pain that is felt is caused by tightness of the fascia and feedback from the mechanoreceptors.

The *heel spur* is a bony protuberance at the bottom of the heel bone and can be seen in an x-ray. When looking closely at the heel spur in the x-ray shown here, we can see that the spur is located precisely where the plantar fascia originates. We can basically attribute the spur to the same cause as hallux valgus, because the extreme tightness of the tendons creates more stress and strain, causing the origin of the plantar fascia to react by getting larger. However, the spur

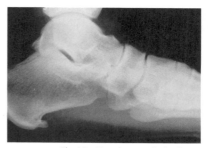

Fig. 17: X-ray image of a heel spur

itself is not the problem but the result of extreme tension and a lack of tendon elasticity. The tendon must therefore be relaxed and gradually lengthened. A foot that is neither resting in a bed nor supported uses the entire tendon when it moves. Loading causes the longitudinal and transverse arches to drop lower, and the tendon lengthens. When the arches are unloaded, the tendon shortens again. That means regular loading and unloading of the naked foot would be an adequate remedy instead of fighting the spur with cortisone and shockwaves.

In addition to acting as a shock absorber, the plantar tendon along with the Achilles tendon has other advantages that can be attributed to the elastic properties of the connective tissue's collagen fibers. Efficient running uses the contractile muscle elements only minimally during a movement, i.e. it uses relatively little oxygen and instead makes maximum use of collagen's elastic springiness. We again need the sensation, strength, and particularly elasticity, but it takes 6-24 months to renew architectural collagen tissue to generate the full potential of our feet.

27 HALLUX VALGUS

The anatomy of the foot shows that the toes are spread, meaning the foot is wide in front and narrow at the heel bone. The exceptional adaptability of the hunter-gatherer, which we retained, is both a blessing and a curse. Much like sitting is the new smoking, shoes are the equivalent of intensive secondhand smoking. Confined to a shoe the foot has no choice but to adapt, and since the shoe has little to nothing to do with the shape of our feet, the foot finally adapts to the shape of the shoe.

The change to the big toe and the connected structures is a huge problem here. Hallux valgus, the crooked big toe, is still dismissed as a hereditary condition but is actually the toe's reaction to being confined to a cage unsuitable for the species. Unless specifically mentioned in the last will and testament, hallux valgus cannot be inherited. The mechanical pressure of a shoe that is too tight pushes the big toe towards the smaller toes for hours a day, seven days a week, causing it to become crooked. This change to its track results in a deviation of the metatarsophalangeal joint, which is then no longer properly loaded. Where the toe was once able to generate and transfer pressure, the joint is now stressed with every step. Much like our palms react to pressure by forming calluses, the joint strengthens itself by adding material, and thus reacting to the increased pressure. The continual stress and strain make it worse until a bunion is clearly visible and the big toe nearly displaces the small ones.

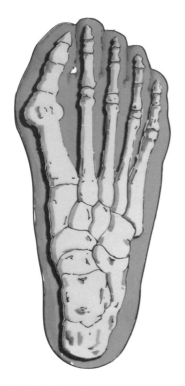

This largely esthetic problem also has functional consequences. The big toe as a stabilizer and initiator at the end of the leg's kinetic chain gradually relinquishes its function, forcing our foundation to lose stability. Try it by standing on one leg and lifting your toes. The disrupted transfer of force to the ground results in another compensatory action, meaning other structures take over the job of the big toe. The muscles of the calf and thigh must compensate for the lack of force transfer with more muscle effort. We know the result: overloading and improper use lead to pain and injury.

Fig. 18: Hallux valgus

During my time as a tennis instructor, I used to watch this spectacle on the adjacent tennis court on Friday evenings. Four gentlemen would arrive after us for a game of doubles. The court was reserved for 8 pm, but the game wouldn't start until 8:30 because they first had to put on all of their bandages and braces. Ankles, knees, and elbows were supported, guided, and sufficiently protected, and yet I could hear them later in the clubhouse complaining about aching feet, knees, and hips.

In addition to the clearly visible supports, they of course wore the appropriate tennis shoes that, like almost all athletic shoes, were equipped with so-called *pronation support*. The same is often boosted with special athletic insoles.

This is usually preceded by a thorough analysis on the treadmill at a sporting goods store or orthopedist's office, who then certify the widely spread over-pronation.

But when we take a closer look at human locomotion, we can see that pronation and even over-pronation isn't a medical condition but an important and natural link in the chain of sub-impulses of the human gait. In simplified terms, the human gait consists of four successive sub-movements, starting with flexing the foot (dorsal flexion). Next, the heel gently makes contact with the ground and the foot tilts to the out-side (supination) and is planted, immediately followed by rolling off to the inside (pronation) and down towards the big toe (plantar flexion). The frequently propagated forefoot strike is of course similar to jogging or Nordic walking.

The pronation that is necessary for efficient propulsion only becomes over-pronation when the stabilizing element, the big toe, leaves its hereditary position and as a result loses its support function. However, it is completely unable to provide support when it is contained inside a modern shoe.

But the response by orthopedists and shoe manufacturers, namely in regards to the pronation support, is unable to adequately replace this function, inevitably making it worse. Like a bouncer, the support doesn't differentiate the good from bad pronation but instead just doesn't allow any pronation. But when the inward movement of the ankle created by Mother Nature, evolution, or God, is missing from the complex motion sequence, the higher-up structures must compensate.

In a nutshell this means, if there is no longer any pronation in the ankle the next joint must pronate, even though the knee hates pronation. This results in meniscus problems, cartilage damage, and cruciate ligament problems that are not just seen in joggers, but increasingly in all soled, active zoo-humans.

But orthopedics, conventional medicine, and medical technology have also found an answer to this. After corrective surgery, a massive knee brace holds the knee joint in place to keep it from pronating.

But cross-joint kinetic chains and fascial structures don't care about bandages. They want to move and in this case, pronate. So when the ankle can no longer pronate because of orthotics, and the knee can no longer pronate because of the brace, who is going to pronate?

On the next floor up, the hip joint and SIJ are looking forward to pronation that should have happened long ago, but the big toe couldn't pronate, so the strain finally rests with the hip where it has no business. After the knee, hip surgery is next and what is much worse is that this unnecessary surgery is the prognosis for the future.

Just like a house, the foundation must be level and sound before the walls can go up. Repairs to floors one and two are only successful if the foundation is strong.

28 FLAT FEET, FALLEN ARCHES, SPLAYFEET

A major area of orthopedic diagnostics is dedicated to labeling the foot as *flat*, having *fallen arches*, or *splayfoot*. When asked about foot problems, many people will mention flat feet. But not because they actually are flat, but rather because they seem flat.

The foot appears flat when it over-pronates. *Pronation* is one of the foot's many movement abilities. They are comprised of the movement abilities of the ankle, which forms the pivot point between the horizontal foot and the vertical rest of the body, and is divided into:

- Upper ankle (tibiofibular fork): lifting and lowering (flexion and extension),

- Lower ankle (talus, heel bone, scaphoid, cuboid),

- Movement abilities in toe joints, bending and extending movements, possibly spreading apart.

Pronation of the foot is a natural shock absorbing motion and a natural internal rotation. This rotation of the foot on its vertical axis, with the outside edge of the foot lifted and the inside edge of the foot lowered without movement of the heel is not only natural but absolutely necessary to keep the biomechanics of the entire leg efficient and injury-free. This pronation is also called internal rotation or inward tilt. The peroneus brevis muscle is primarily responsible for pronation of the foot. So-called overpronation causes the edge of the foot to tilt heavily inward, loading the ligaments, tendons, and joints. This overpronation can have various causes, but is usually caused by the missing big toe, or more precisely, the displaced big toe. Because instead of providing stability in its hereditary position as an extension of the first metatarsophalangeal joint, it has been pushed over towards its little brothers. Misalignment of the foot, or excess weight, or extreme fatigue exacerbates the absence of the big toe and intensifies the arch collapse.

As a general rule, excessive pronation as well as flat feet and fallen arches can be attributed to inadequate functioning of the adjoining muscles. Shoes will show heavy wear in the medial area (usually the inside). Overpronation stemming from the heavy wear can be controlled with supports or supporting elements. But this intervention changes the complete biomechanics long-term, permanently overloading the knees and hips even while only standing.

Underpronation or *supination* is more rare. The tilting of the foot to its outside edge, the opposite of pronation, is only possible with the lazy soles of athletic shoes. The raised heel and massive rubber edge form the raised center of gravity and lever, allowing the ankle to roll outward. The fear of rolling an ankle and the associated supination trauma are what cause people to use braces and athletic tape. These are supposed to support the foot and prevent the rolling, i.e. tearing of the lateral collateral ligaments. But the lack of stability is in fact not improved by the use of braces. Instead, the foot is further robbed of its natural abilities, and eventually loses them.

Upon closer examination, particularly when standing on the commercial pressure measurement plate also used by orthopedists, the flat foot is no longer a flat foot. During a simplified analysis, the pressure measurement plate's software shows what the imprint of a flat foot should look like, and the affected individuals are usually shocked when what they see and what the flat foot model looks like are not at all the same. Most feet are less flat than previously thought, and are only atrophied. That means the muscles necessary for an upright position as well as the elasticity have declined so much that the foot is flat. When you don't water a potted plant for an extended period of time, its leaves and blooms will begin to droop. But as soon as you start to regularly water it again, they straighten up.

Most of the time those affected have been wearing orthotics for years, and more often than that they have already disposed of them after a few months, or in some cases simply stopped using them. The orthotic is supposed to stabilize and support the flat foot, which although is well intended, is in fact not good for it.

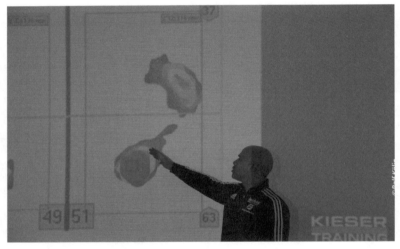

Typical footprint without the big toe on a pressure measurement plate

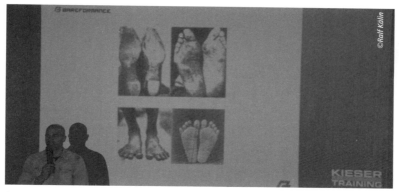

Comparison of normal and natural feet

Let's imagine we are in a room where the ceiling is no longer sound and is at risk of collapse. In our desperation, we go to the hardware store for advice. We leave the hardware store with a bunch of supports and place them under the ceiling. We return a year later to check if the ceiling has become sounder, but against our expectation, that is not the case. The clerk at the hardware store suggests buying new hydraulic, laser-guided supports at many times the price of the basic supports, and we buy them and wait another year to come back and check the ceiling's soundness again.

An orthotic is no more able to make the arch capable of bearing weight than the support beams. It merely takes over the function instead of restoring it. A flat foot, and experts agree on this, is caused by a lack of muscle strength and a lack of elastic fascial structures to support the arch and hold it up. Thus the solution can only lie in the use, the training, of active structures, ideally in their original state, namely barefoot.

29 FOREST FLOOR GOOD, ASPHALT BAD

The popular belief that we should only run on a soft forest floor or at the beach is as absurd as believing in the magical properties of plastic foam soles. People like to believe they are protecting their joints when they run on a soft surface, in our climates preferably on soft forest soil.

Some avoid asphalt like the plague and blame it on the myriad of pains and injuries that result from habitual jogging, instead of questioning the manner in which they recklessly jump from one heel to the other. In some cases, the fear of asphalt is so great that people will run on the narrow strip of grass and hazard the hidden dog turds and holes.

The fact is, while asphalt isn't natural, it isn't much harder than a beaten track in nature and it also challenges and fosters our feet's natural abilities. Our feet are perfectly equipped for shock absorption. A unique system of muscles and tendons allow the foot to not only absorb the bulk of the impact with the plantar and Achilles tendons' elasticity, but also recycle it for propulsion.

The rule of thumb is: the harder the surface, the greater the reaction forces, much like a ball that is bounced on the floor.

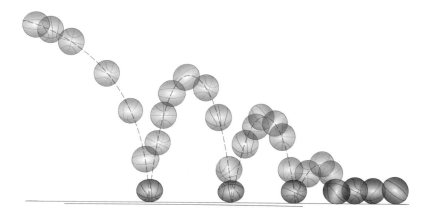

Fig. 19: Elasticity

30 ATHLETE'S FOOT

The ambivalent relationship between people and their feet is rooted in the fact that the latter rarely receive the attention that they deserve.

First thing in the morning, they are shut away and forced to endure housing conditions that would infuriate any animal rights activist.

Too tight, no daylight, no activity, and a lack of fresh air. In some cases, the result disgusts us to the point where some people feel queasy at the sight of naked feet. Most people consider their feet ugly and here foot care is just a drop in the bucket.

If a manicured hand is our calling card, the foot is the disabled, pallid and hunchbacked brother Quasimodo leading a miserable existence in the cellar. That's why not taking off your socks and sandals even at the beach isn't so bad and definitely understandable. And those who bravely release their naked feet into the hostile environment are met with shards of glass, nails, sharp stones, and particularly funguses that are just waiting to attack us.

The myth that pedestrians cannot walk barefoot in cities without getting injured is widespread. But the reality looks quite different, and most walking paths and pedestrian zones are truly refuges for pure bipedalism if one walks with the necessary awareness and eyes on the ground.

The awareness in particular will set in as soon as you have taken off your shoes and your feet are able to feel the ground beneath them.

People consider fungal infections of the feet a constant danger to their health.

In fact, a foot fungus only flourishes under certain conditions. Like many fungus species, foot fungus also requires a moist and warm climate such as that of an indoor swimming pool or sauna. What is interesting is that foot fungus is less of a problem outdoors such as in an outdoor swimming pool. This appearance is not deceptive, in fact moisture alone is not enough so if there isn't sufficient warmth or it is too hot, a foot fungus will not thrive.

While foot fungus is often contracted at an indoor pool, the fungus only begins to develop inside the shoe. Here the shoe takes on the function of an incubator. Any remaining moisture between the toes, combined with the warmth inside the shoe allows the fungus to bloom, and an initial itching heralds its imminent appearance. Without shoes, a foot fungus is practically useless. A sweaty foot condition also cannot be found with bare feet. Although feet do sweat without shoes, the smell is not as pungent. You get a similar affect when you wear polyester shirts while exercising.

Working out in socks or barefoot at the fitness studio is thus more of an esthetic than hygiene issue. In general, the naked foot is not a threat to our health. Germs and bacteria must come into contact with mucous membranes, and in that regard the surface of the hand, presents a much greater danger.

31 BAREFOOT & SHOES

An oxymoron is a rhetorical figure of speech that is comprised of two opposing or mutually exclusive terms. For example, like liquid gas or love-hate relationship, barefoot is also an oxymoron.

The supply of so-called barefoot shoes is overseeable, but the major hype has passed. The market-dominating sporting goods manufacturers have more or less dismissed this special interest sector, or never entered it in the first place. A few supposedly small labels are courageously standing their ground.

Yet there is an assortment of barefoot shoes available to consumers online or on the shelves of the plastic foam wonderland.

The Vibram Five Fingers is a particularly bizarre epitome of the barefoot shoe species. This shoe combines some positive characteristics with a design that unmistakably says: "I am barefoot."

The design includes a cone for each toe, making the shoe look less like a shoe and more like a bare foot enveloped in a fitted, sensible shell for the foot and its toes.

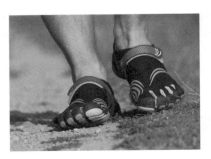

Yet throughout human history and the associated fashion faux pas, no one has had the terrific idea to construct shoes with a separate cone for each toe. Samurai and Ninja footwear have soles that separate the big toe from the other toes, and the sandals of the Tarahumara also separate only the big toe from the smaller toes.

And there is a simple reason for that. Just like during recess when we were children, the big guy, the big toe, likes to stand independently and confidently in the schoolyard, controlling the action. The little guys, and especially the little toes, like to be together. There is strength in numbers so they stand together and share their snacks. If one of the little guys leaves the group, thereby changing the dynamics, the others get nervous and search for community and safety within the group.

In terms of anatomy, the small toes utilize one tendon and one muscle strand to move the sensory contact to each other. That is the reason they cannot move independent of each other and always react as a group. Therefore, it makes little sense to mechanically separate the contact of the toes to each other and place them in solitary confinement, when they thrive and much prefer the group dynamics.

The little toes become stressed because as herd animals, they are now on their own and can no longer cooperate. The result is that the small toes' important ability to help the big toe permanently maintain balance is severely impaired, just like a canoe with an outrigger that becomes unstable when the outrigger is gone.

The sensation, meaning the ability to create balance, is impaired by the stress produced by the separation of the toes. It has been proven that the ability to balance while standing on one leg is quite good, whereas changing to Vibram Five Fingers worsens the ability to balance similar to jogging shoes.

It is also interesting that the toe cones form a larger surface overall that consequently releases more heat, or rather allows the foot to become hypothermic more quickly. The toes can no longer warm each other. That is also why mittens keep the hands warmer than gloves. So if you like cold feet, you should choose toe cones.

Something that is also of note is that after running together, the runners wearing Five Fingers always took much longer to get dressed after an exercise unit than anyone else. Placing each toe in individual shells simply takes more effort, especially since we don't all have the same toes. But the shells assume that we do, therefore offering the same cones regardless of the individual differences in our toes when it comes to length and width.

No matter how many people love and value them, foot beds also make little sense. Sleep deprivation in feet is virtually unknown, so a foot that has gone to sleep is as desirable as a flat tire. But the fact that there is a bed for every kind of foot, should cause us to pause. How could it be possible that our feet, which are basically constructed the same way but with definite differences with respect to details and shape of individual structures, can all use one and the same foot bed? The idea would be praiseworthy if the foot bed was individualized and quasi customized, however the foot bed is devoid of any logic.

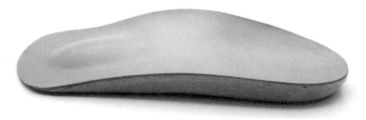

32 SHOES THAT MAKE SENSE

The first thing we do at the end of a long day on our feet is take off our shoes and put up our feet. And with good reason, since our feet in particular are generally inappropriately housed in tight and sloped footwear. The perfect shoe, be it for running or everyday wear, or for the office, should not restrict the foot and allow it to function as if it were barefoot. Furthermore, its sensory function should be enabled along with protection of as much sole as possible, and as much sensation as possible.

The following criteria should be considered:

Sensory function and feedback: much like a car that continuously gathers information with its wheels in order to be able to intervene in extreme situations with a stabilization program and ABS, we are also dependent on the flawless transfer of data from the ground that we walk on. It is the job of our feet to do so, and shoes should not impede them.

Protection: the sensitive sole of the foot must be protected, even if it senses some things early with the appropriate sensory function. I noticed that I step on fewer Legos when I walk through my children's rooms barefoot, or at least get a warning from my foot at the slightest contact which then prevents me from setting it down. The sole should protect the foot from injury from things like thorns, etc., and should also provide some protection against heat and cold.

Shape and last: the last, which is the shoe's outline, must correspond to the anatomy of the foot and not vice versa. The foot is wide in front and narrow in the back, which can be seen without intensive anatomical study. In the same way that a jacket has two sleeves, or pants have two legs so that they will fit us, the shape of shoes should correspond to that of the foot. Since the foot spreads under weight, the pointy toe and generally raised toe box should be avoided even if it is the latest fashion. However, the look of a shoe with a wide toe box requires some getting used to.

Heel and lift: from a biomechanical point of view, the heel that used to help a rider into his stirrups, lifting the noble ladies and gentlemen above the common folk as befitted their social class, has completely outlived its usefulness and no longer has a purpose other than providing some relief to joggers who are continuously jumping on their heels. You should therefore forgo heels. However, if you like to jog and enjoy jumping on your heels, please wear running shoes with a cushioned heel.

Support and cushioning: less is more, especially when it comes to the technological achievements regarding Gel, Boost, Shot and Air. Cushioning doesn't mean you can jump off your garage and land safely. And the much lauded energy retrieval that would launch you back to the top of your garage with one jump, is a downright lie. In reality, we are talking about energy-directing wedges under our soles, because plastic foam et al. cushions primarily force transfer to the ground, and much like a basketball you bounce on a soft gym mat after first bouncing it on a hard gym floor, you will notice that it takes much more energy to bounce the ball the same way.

The right footwear is critical to strong feet. A shoe model named *Free* does not necessarily imply freedom for your feet. It is more like Light Cola that also doesn't necessarily make it easier to lose weight. As with a diet, it doesn't help if you work out every day, but your first stop after removing your shoes is the refrigerator.

Therefore, the rule of thumb is to wear shoes with plenty of toe room and no heel as often as possible. Much like your body during a hard strength workout, your feet will let you know when they have had enough, and you should listen. Also try occasionally taking off your shoes when you are away from home. The next time you are out walking in suitable terrain, like on a sidewalk, just go barefoot and then put your shoes back on. Just don't overdo it!

And finally, it is important to train the feet. Below are some tips on this subject.

33 PLASTIC FOAM REHAB

After the foray through our developmental history and a look through the lens of the laws of nature based on physics, biology, and lots of common sense, some orthopedic myths should have lost their splendor and the hardware-software incompatibility should have been conveyed. It's not about differentiating right from wrong, pointing fingers, or pinning blame on someone.

Rather, it is a plea, an encouraging nudge to fundamentally change your awareness of your feet. But be careful not to overreact. If you now throw away your running shoes out of indignation or enthusiasm and run 6 miles barefoot around the lake, you will likely feel even less enjoyment than during your usual runs. Like working out or practicing, the progression should be from easy to complex in accordance to the principles of training theory. In this context, the movement hierarchy provides us with the perfect blueprint for relearning our abilities. Just like we once learned to move as children, standing, then walking, then running.

You have taken the first step.

- Try to relieve your feet of shoes as often as possible. Thick socks can usually substitute slippers.

- Whether at home or under your desk, there are always things you can pick up with your feet, lift, or use to roll along the sole of your foot.

- Purchase some species-appropriate footwear with lots of room for your toes, without heels, and with very little cushioning.

- Wear these shoes occasionally. If you wear them for too long, meaning too much freedom, strain, and activity, your feet will usually answer with noticeable irritation.

- Don't overdo it! A short walk or outing is often not a problem for untrained feet, but take along an old pair of shoes in case your feet do start to complain.

- Stick with short intervals. Standing and walking are the perfect training for your soles.

- Combine the weight-bearing activity of standing and walking with exercises in this book to add additional stimuli and minimize pain via fascia exercises.

If that goes well and there aren't any problems, try increasing your walks and occasionally taking off your barefoot shoes. A few yards on the sidewalk or in a parking lot are sufficient. You should be sufficiently aware of the ground to avoid stepping on rocks or broken glass.

Running, and doing so without shoes, is something you should only reconsider after appropriate coaching. Contrary to the opinion of some coaches, it can be learned in a class setting. But experience shows that the successful changeover is a process that has to be properly maintained long-term.

34 BACKWARDS IS THE NEW FORWARDS

We can hardly go higher, faster, and farther. Our striving for top performances or for avoiding any physical activity is boundless. The middle of the road is no longer en vogue. Yet we are neither the strongest nor the fastest creatures on the planet, but are mediocre and quite good at it. Perhaps this is the reason that we crave the extreme. We are not really good at one thing, but kind of good at everything.

It is exciting that the number of fitness studios and fitness instructors increases every year, but it does not seem to have any effect on the number of people suffering from back, knee, or shoulder pain. Quite the opposite is true in fact. The 19 attractive European establishments with their seductively large assortment of high-quality machines offer satisfaction for the broad and less broad masses.

It seems a piece of the puzzle is missing and the statement: "a strong back feels no pain," requires more nuanced consideration.

Something is going wrong. The human body depends on the flawless function of the sole of the foot, and problems with the foundation also cause problems on the first and second floor.

This hardware-software incompatibility is not simply solved with strong feet. Just like shoes force our feet into an unhealthy relieving posture, chairs have the same effect on knees, hips, lumbar spine, and shoulder girdle.

Not only have we forgotten how to stand, but we have also forgotten our heritage. It is important to understand that "barefoot" is not a trend but was the basis for our evolution and has carried our feet for millions of years throughout history. It is therefore time for us to give our feet more attention again. More precisely, we should develop more awareness of our foundation because attention is all too quickly diverted.

35 RUNNING RELOAD

The civilized human neglects his feet based on the motto "out of sight, out of mind," and allows the soles of his feet to become woefully stunted. Before a human is even able to walk, he is already outfitted with shoes as an infant.

People that live in a natural way and usually don't or rarely wear shoes are just as skilled with their toes as they are with their hands. Flat feet, fallen arches, or splayfoot are unknown or undetected since there are no orthopedists nearby.

Wearing shoes regularly prevents the foot from actively participating in the movement and from developing abilities based on "form follows function." Abilities even deteriorate and the foot becomes stunted to the point of being unable to move without shoes. Once caught up in this dependency, flip-flops become obligatory at the beach even though it is warm enough and there is no risk of injury in the pool area.

Joggers and runners must therefore begin by training their feet, strengthening them and making them more flexible so that stunted soles can redevelop.

According to the hierarchy of movement to do so, the easiest exercise, standing, must be practiced first.

When we relinquish our toes, we are left with only three muscles to facilitate forward movement (peronaeus longus, peronaeus brevis, and tibialis posterior).

The remaining muscles then feed into the phalanges. Next to the muscles at the sole of the foot, they are the large calf muscles that feed into the Achilles tendon, as well as the long toe flexors that come from the calf. Thus toe training will exercise the sole of the foot as well as a large portion of the calf muscles.

36 FOOT EXERCISES

FUNCTIONALITY BEGINS WITH THE FEET

Training concepts and trends regarding strength and endurance come and go, and our feet take part in all of them. The fitness industry offers classes and strength training, be it in a circuit or with free weights, and of course endurance training on the treadmill, bicycle ergometer, or cross trainer, all with the presumption that we are good walkers. Every movement, every sport, every workout is based on the flawless function of our feet and the associated stability of the superior joints and muscles, from the ankles to the hips. When this flawless function is already impaired at the foundation and at the interface and transfer area to the ground, errors and problems happen automatically. The result of this is pain.

ON SOLID GROUND

There is a machine to work practically every muscle, but the sole of the foot and the fascial structures are simply ignored, wasting away in plastic foam. A house is only as solid as its foundation, a tree only as strong as its roots, but the modern man completely forgets his feet.

It is time that we pay more attention to our feet and make them strong and flexible again.

INFORMATION ABOUT THE IMPLEMENTS

Some exercises include the use of loop bands, a medicine ball, or a stability trainer. A well-equipped fitness studio has lots of equipment. The exercises with and without small implements can easily be done at home. The implements are important to the exercises in order to train the stability and sensory motor skills of the feet.

Toebility offers solutions for the following symptoms:

- Tired feet and balance problems

- Fallen arches, flat feet, splayfoot

- Bunions

- Inflammation of the Achilles tendon

- Meniscus irritation

- ISJ blockage

- Heel spurs

- Morton's neuroma

- Hallux rigidus

- Shin splints

- Patella irritation

GENERAL PREPARATION FOR THE EXERCISES:

After every exercise, check your big toe, meaning press the big toe into the ground and lift your small toes. It should get increasingly easier.

1. Stand comfortably and press your big toe firmly into the ground while simultaneously lifting the small toes. It sounds simple, but can be difficult especially in the beginning. Start out slow and gradually increase the effort with each repetition. It is important to keep the ball of the foot on the floor during the exercise so don't lift the entire foot when you try to raise your toes. As soon as your proprioception improves, you can hold this position for up to 30 seconds.

2. Curl your big toe under your foot. You can use your hands if necessary. This movement can be unpleasant (often with a limited range of motion), which is why it is important that you do this exercise on a soft surface. During this movement, the emphasis should be placed on the mobility of the first metatarsal bone. When looking down from above, it will look like the big toe has been chopped off.

3. Bend the four small toes under your foot with or without your hands so only the big toe points forward. Now press your big toe into the ground to reinforce this position. This exercise, too, should be performed on a soft surface because bending the toes can be unpleasant. This exercise works on metatarsal mobility.

START OF TRAINING

Please be sure to take your time with the individual exercises and do them gently. You should also avoid overloading by training too often and too intensively.

It is assumed that these exercises will be performed barefoot as this has already been mentioned several times throughout this book..

Starting position:

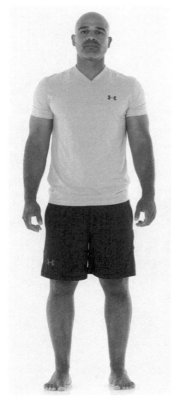
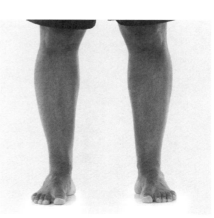

EXERCISE 1 – BIG TOE DOWN

Begin by reinitiating contact with your toes. This is important because permanently wearing shoes limits the functioning of the feet. The specific purpose is to improve the foot musculature, as well as increase the mobility of participating joints. This exercise serves as an easy first step and an initial contact.

a)   Grip the floor with your five toes. Hold this position for 20 seconds and then release.

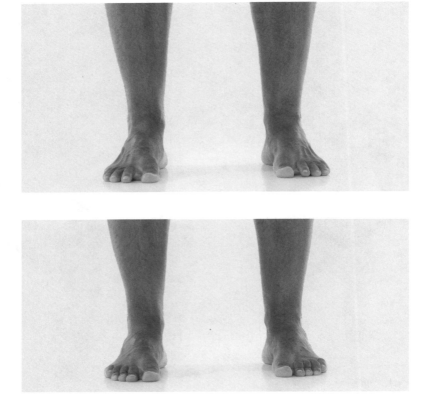

A different angle:

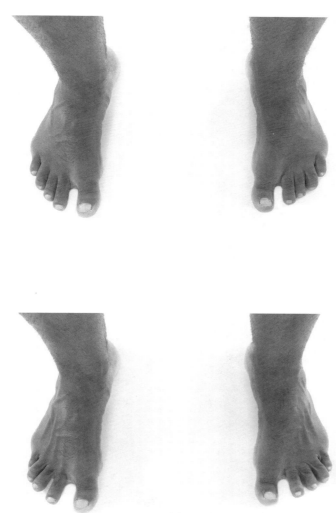

b) Now press your big toe into the floor while simultaneously lifting the small toes. Here you initially practice control of the big toe, then mobility, and finally work the muscles of the big toe.

Please note: keep the leg straight during the exercise and don't bend the ankle!

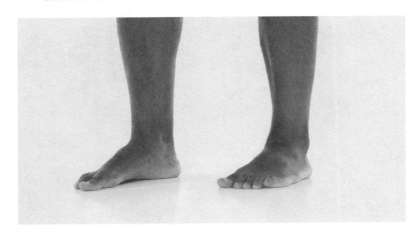

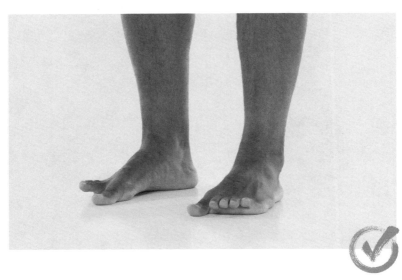

Please note: this is the **wrong** way to do the exercise.

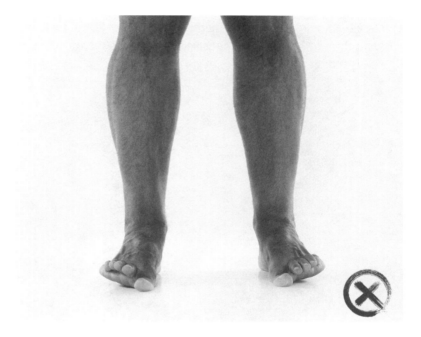

EXERCISE 2 – BIG TOE MOBILITY I

a) Stand on one leg and bend the toes of the other leg under (back) and then add some slight pressure. Hold this position for 20 seconds and then switch feet.

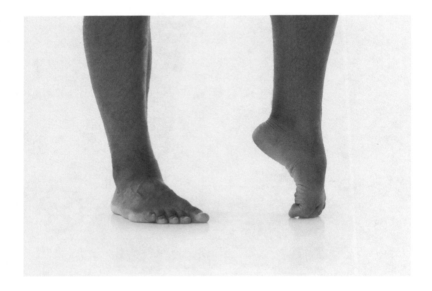

The goal of this exercise is to work on extension of the ankle as well as flexion of the metatarsophalangeal joint of the big toe in the muscle chain.

Please note: if you have a stiff metatarsophalangeal joint such as after bunion surgery, please do this exercise very carefully!

b)   Now fold the small toes back and the big toe forward. Then try to press the big toe into the floor. Hold this position for 20 seconds and then switch feet.

Here again the focus is on the functional separation between the big toe and small toes with respect to strength and mobility.

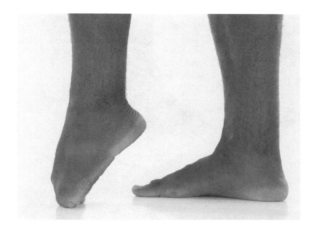

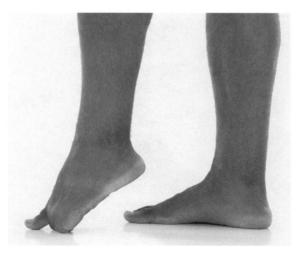

FIT FEET FOR LIFE

Switch sides: right foot

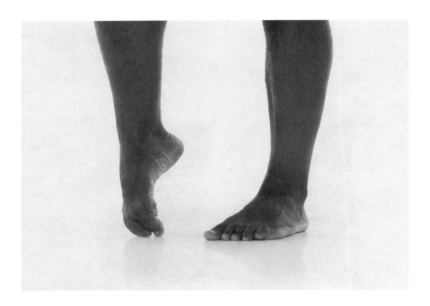

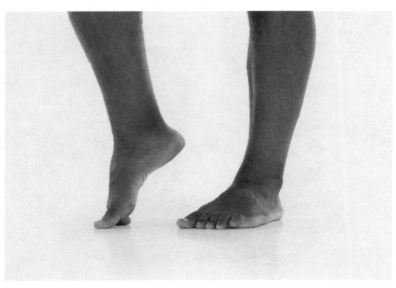

EXERCISE 3 – BIG TOE MOBILITY II

In this exercise, you fold the big toe back. Then try to add moderate pressure with the small toes by pressing them into the floor. This exercise is beneficial because the metatarsophalangeal joint works in both directions, which is why both directions must be practiced.

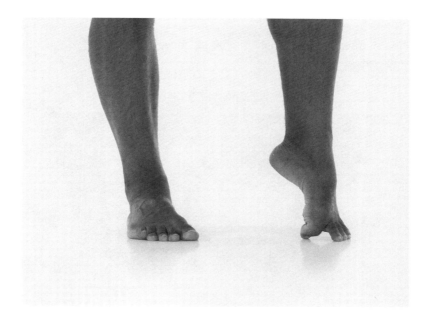

EXERCISE 4 – ABDUCTION/ADDUCTION

Stand so your heels touch but the two metatarsophalangeal joints are approximately half an inch apart. Now try to move the tips of your big toes inward so that they touch. Here we work on abduction and adduction of the metatarsophalangeal joint, or rather lateral movement of the big toe. Overall we are working on the metatarsophalangeal joint's latent mobility.

Please note: make sure only the big toe moves and the ball of the foot stays put!

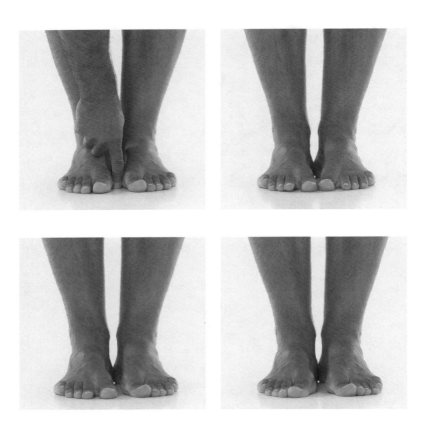

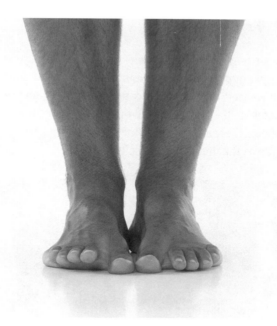

A different angle:

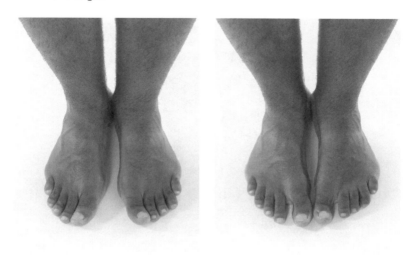

EXERCISE 5 – CATERPILLAR

a) Flex your toes and spread them apart. Then release them to the floor. Next grip the floor with your toes and use all of your strength to pull yourself forward like a caterpillar. Make sure the movement originates in the toes and not the legs or hips. Ideally this exercise should be performed as one motion sequence. This exercise strengthens the muscles of the soles.

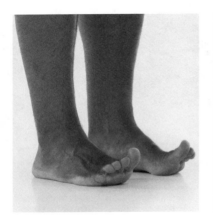 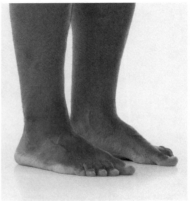

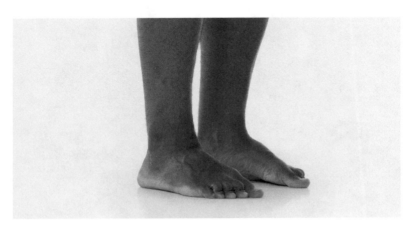

b)   If you are unable to move forward during the original exercise, you can place a towel or a mini stabilizing unit under your heel. However, it is important that your heel doesn't act as a brake during the exercise.

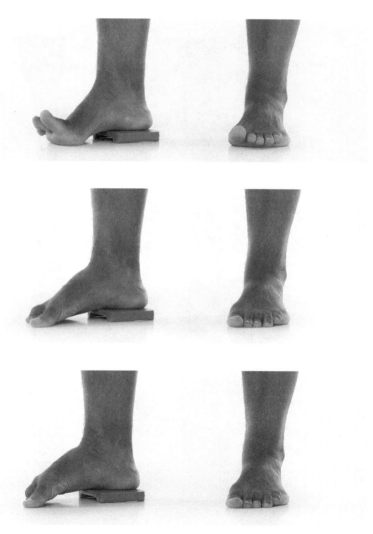

c)   In this variation, you will use an exercise band or even a towel and place it in front of your foot. Now try to move the band or towel with the same toe movement you performed in the previous exercise. Here, too, it is important that the movement originates in the toes.

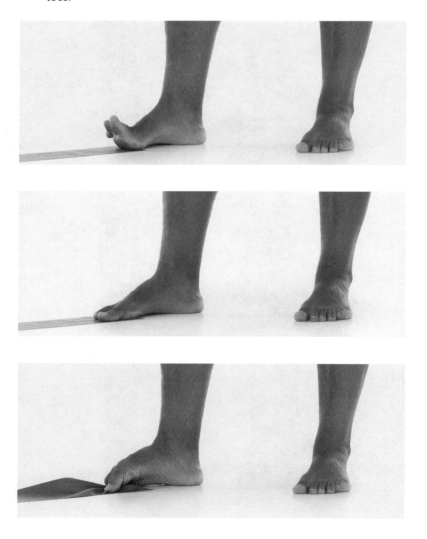

EXERCISE 6 – SITTING ON YOUR HEELS

a)   Get down on your knees and slowly sit back on your heels. Make
      sure your feet are extended.

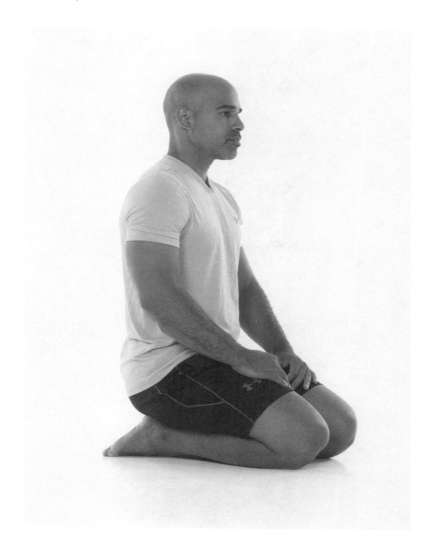

b) Now carefully lean back and support yourself with your hands on the floor behind your back. Now push the pelvis forward and extend the hips. You are now working on ankle extension as well as the entire muscle chain by way of knee flexion and hip extension (rectus femoris, iliopsoas).

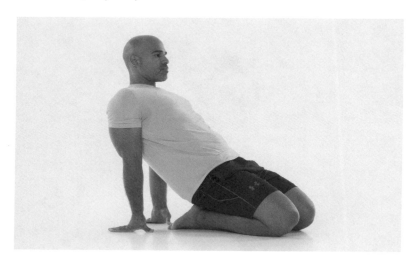

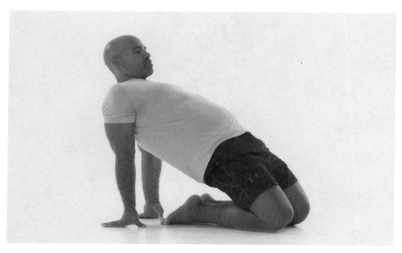

c)   Now repeat exercises a) and b) but tuck your toes and press them into the floor. The pressure of the toes allows you to feel the tension all the way up into the hip flexors. Here, too, you are working the metatarsophalangeal joints of the individual toes.

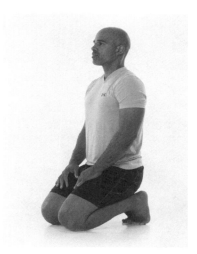 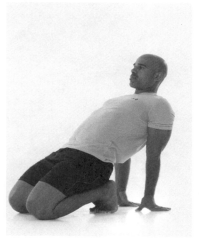

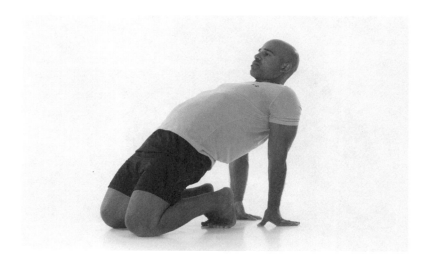

A different angle:

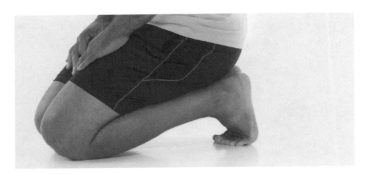

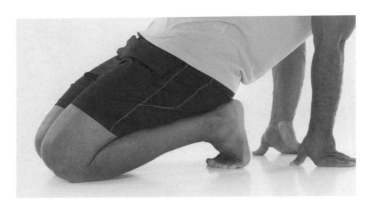

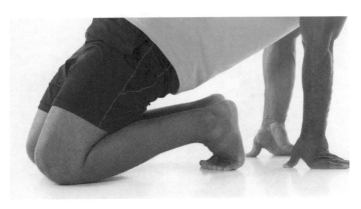

EXERCISE 7 – ADDUCTION/ABDUCTION WITH LOOP + BALL

You will need: a small ball and a loop band

Starting position:
Begin by positioning your foot over a small ball (approx. 1 – 1 ½ inches in diameter).

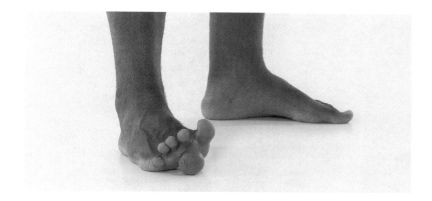

a)   Now try to grip the ball with your toes. This works toe strength and mobility. In this exercise, it does not matter with which toes you grip the ball.

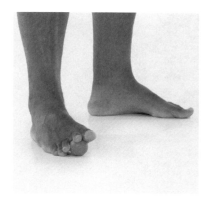 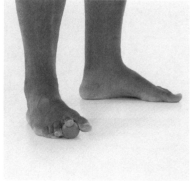

b) Once you have successfully gripped the ball with your toes, try to clamp it between your big toe and the adjacent small toe, and then carefully lift it. This usually works almost automatically.

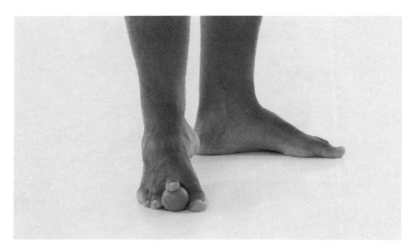

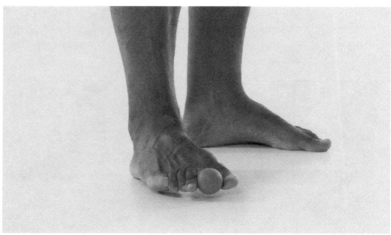

c) For this exercise, stretch the loop band between your two big toes. Now turn your feet out on your heels, adding tension to the band. This works the metatarsophalangeal joints as well as the external rotation of the legs. Make sure the movement originates in the feet and not the knee joints.

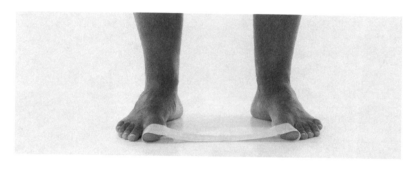

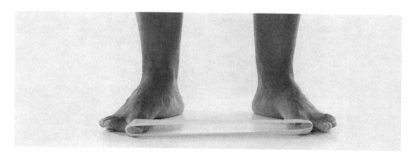

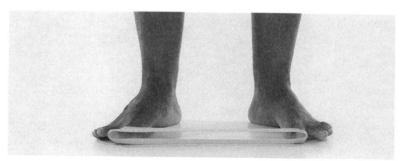

d) This variation focuses on increasing the load by holding one leg in place and only working the other side.

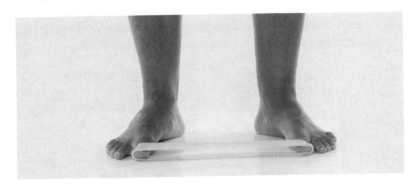

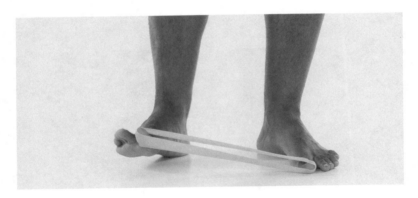

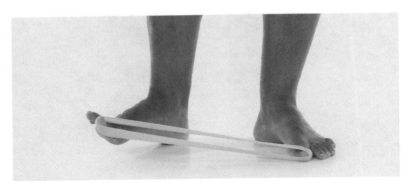

EXERCISE 8 – MINI STABILIZATION TRAINER/ STABILITY BETWEEN PRONATION AND SUPINATION

When working with the mini stabilization trainer (MST), the focus is on coordinating the forefoot and the big toe on the slightly unstable units.

The MST consists of four units that can provide different stimuli when placed on the floor. The idea is to work on ankle activity to train body stability by consciously creating instability in the foot's long and transverse axis.

What you need: tilt board (blue), therapeutic spinning top (red), level board (green)

Starting position:

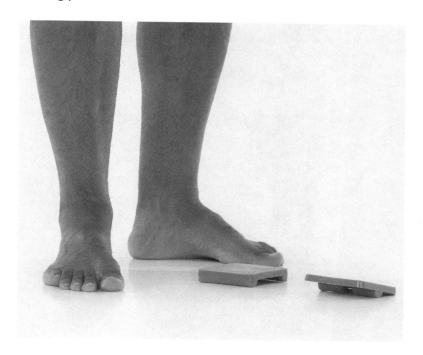

a) Place the level board under your heel and the tilt board under your toes so that the heel is planted on the level board and the forefoot's long axis is unstable on the tilt board (blue). Now slowly lift the other foot and try to balance on the units. The forefoot is now working along its long axis and tries to create stability.

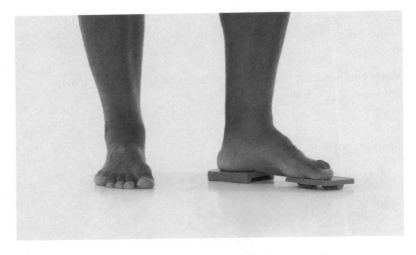

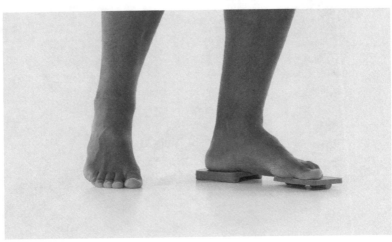

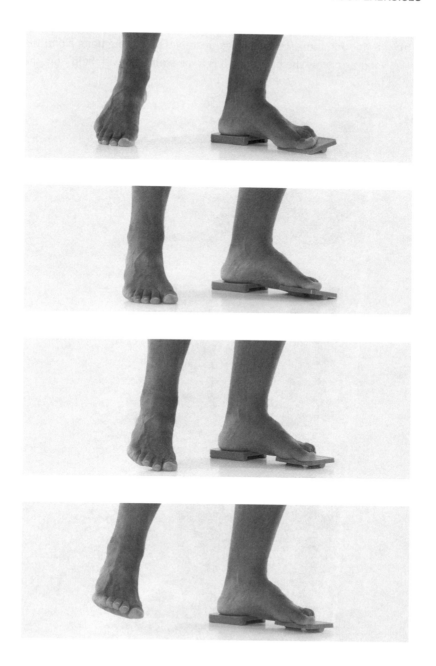

b) In this variation, we switch the unstable and stable units along the long axis. Now the heel bone has to be stabilized with help from the forefoot.

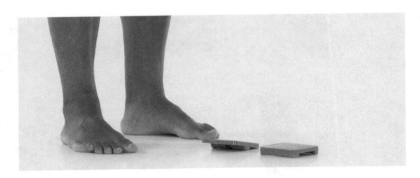

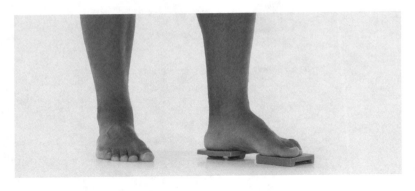

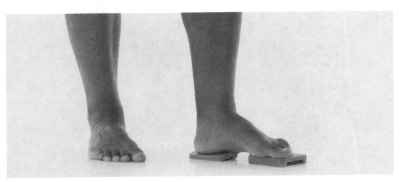

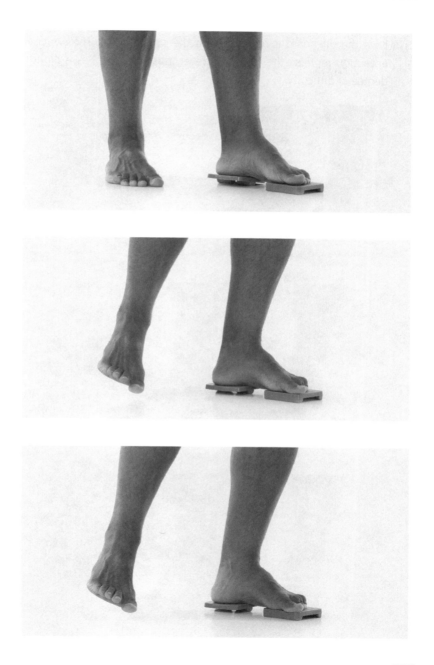

c) Now the tilt board is replaced with the spinning top. The exercise execution remains the same. However, this variation has a higher degree of difficulty.

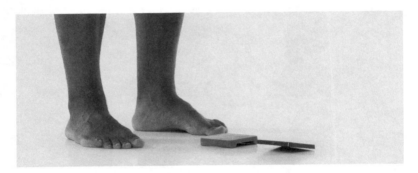

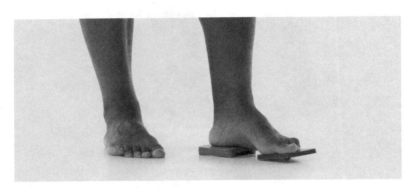

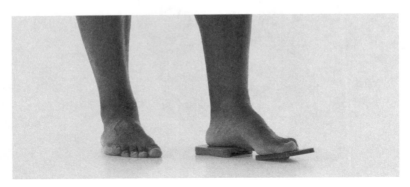

d)   This makes the heel unstable again. See variation b).

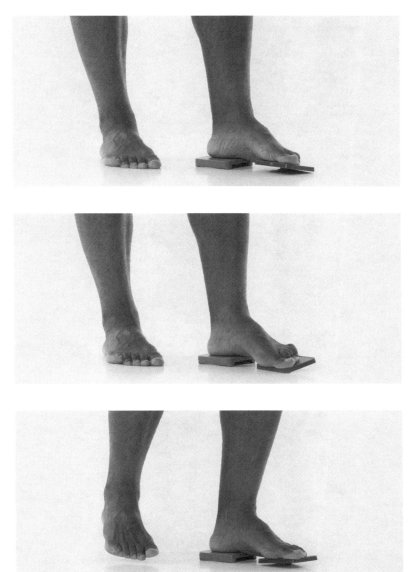

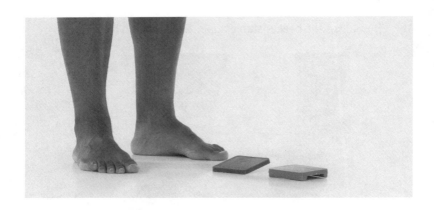

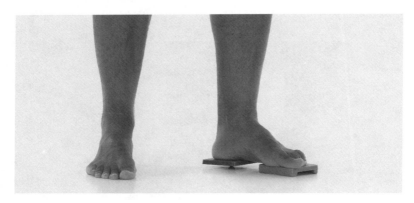

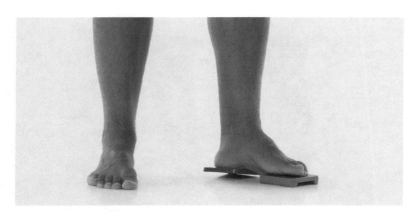

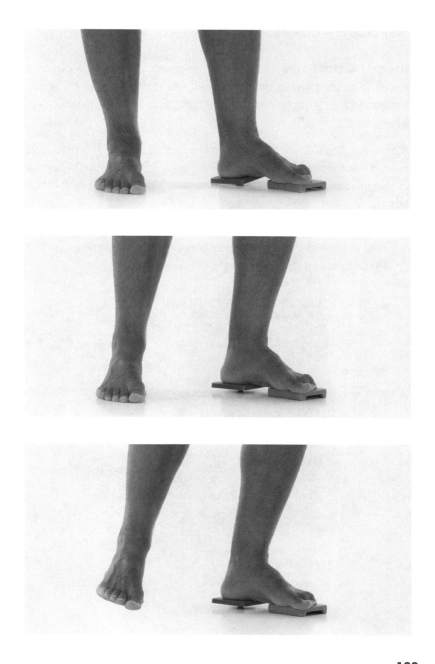

EXERCISE 9 – COMPLEX EXERCISES/WALKING

Now that we have easily and simply performed the standing exercises according to the training theory, we will now implement the previously learned skills in a more complex and difficult way with dynamic processes.

In principal, this exercise sequence focuses on relearning and practicing the four basic movements of the ankle: "flexion" (dorsal flexion), "outside tilt" (supination), "inside tilt" (pronation), and "downward push" (plantar flexion).

a) Pull the toes towards the shin (dorsal flexion) and gently rest the heel in front of the body's center of gravity. Then lower the forefoot to the floor and shift your weight forward.

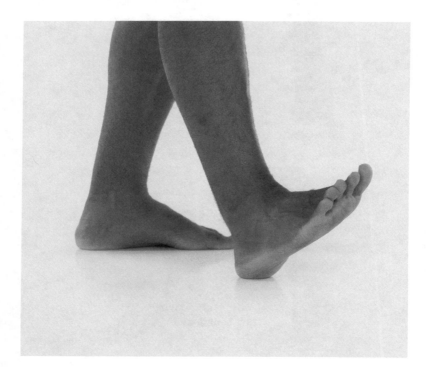

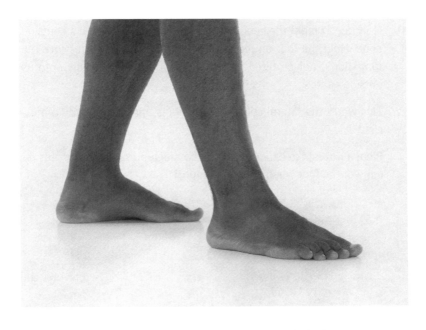

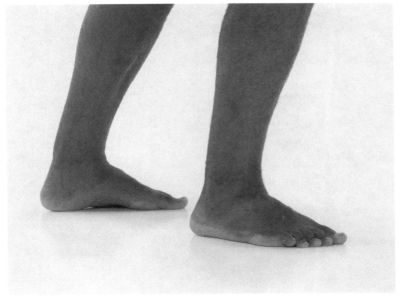

b) Now gently plant the heel, but this time tilt the foot onto its outside edge. Hold the foot on its outside edge and vary the pressure. The foot should not be tilted all the way to the floor but only onto its outside edge.

This works the lateral collateral ligaments and corresponding muscles.

Please note: take care not to put too much pressure on the outside edge of the foot when you roll the foot!

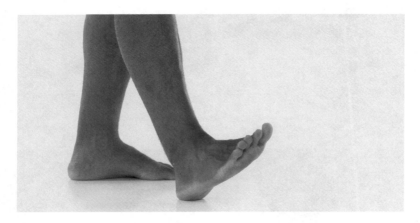

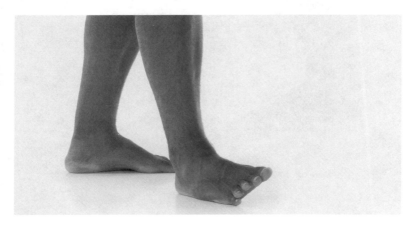

c)   In this exercise, you go from supination (see exercise b) to prona-
     tion. This movement must be actively initiated by the big toe. After
     the foot has been planted on its outside edge, it is actively tilted
     inward.

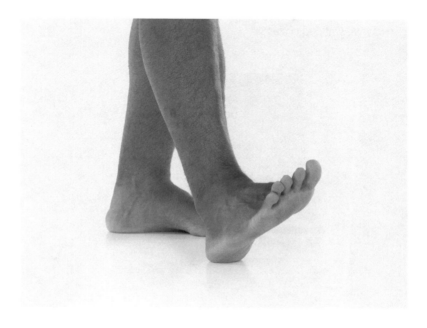

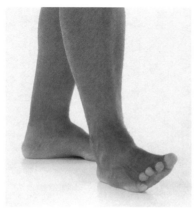

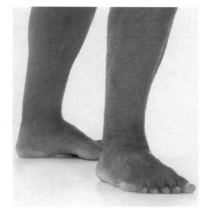

d) In the last exercise of this exercise sequence, we add the final and critical movement, which is pressing the foot into the floor, to the previous flows. This means after dorsal flexion, supination, and pronation, the weight shifts to the forefoot followed by the roll-off onto the toes, and then finally to the big toe. This exercise represents the active walking cycle.

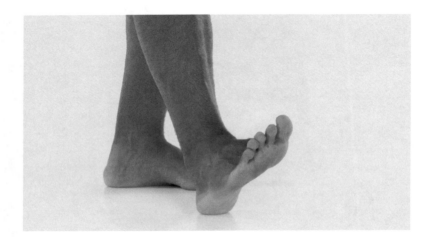

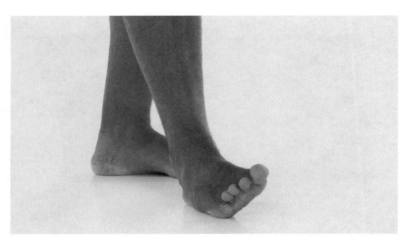

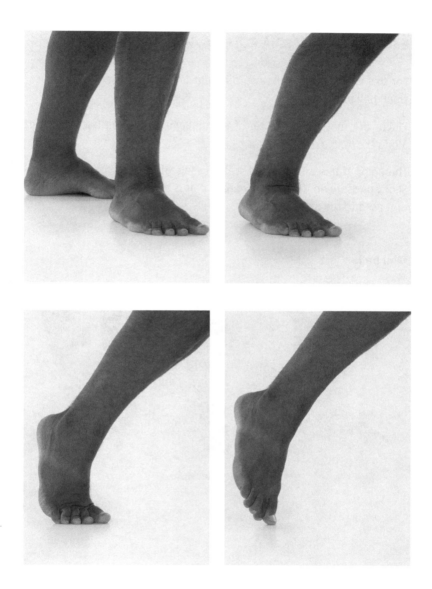

EXERCISE 10 – FASCIA ROLLING/PLANTAR FASCIA

For this exercise, you will need different implements like, for instance, a small ball and a roller.

Place your foot on the center of the implement and roll back and forth along the long axis of the foot.

The point of this exercise is to scan the sole of the foot for painful spots. Slight pressure on the respective pain points as well as the rolling get the foot used to the movement.

Mini ball

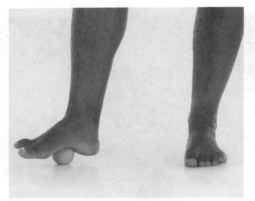
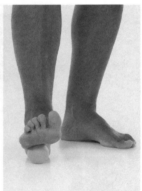

Duoball

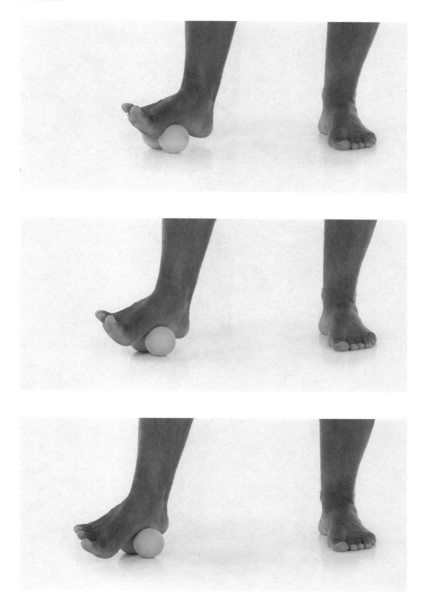

Mini roller

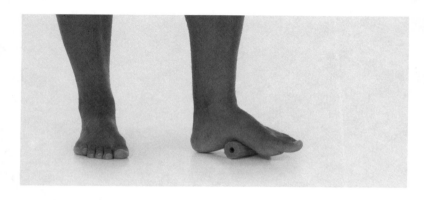

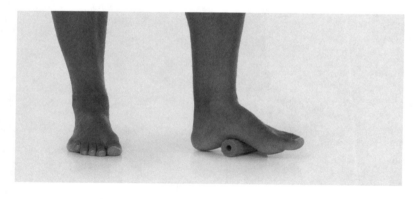

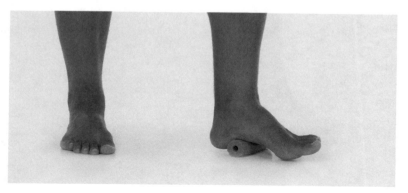

Blackroll mini

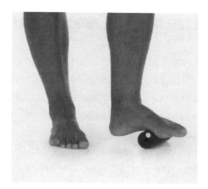

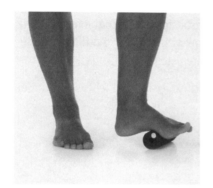

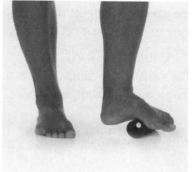

Twister

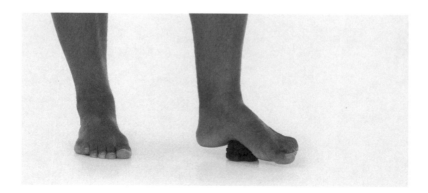

EXERCISE 11 – FASCIA ROLLING/CALF

Fasciae are connective tissue structures that envelop every organ, every ligament and muscle like a thin, delicate skin. They are an organ that completely interlink and structure the entire body. Fasciae should be both firm and elastic. One-sided postures and a lack of exercise can cause them to get sticky and matted. As a result, they lose their elasticity and cause the body to feel stiff. This can lead to discomfort, limitations and physical malaise. Since fasciae maintain the shape of the muscle and protect it from injury, they should absolutely be worked and kept, or rather made, supple. Next to moving and doing the exercises shown in the previous chapter, it is beneficial to transfer stimuli to the fascia in the form of rolling movements and pressure with the aid of different implements like Blackroll® (balls, rollers, twister, etc.).

The focus of this group of fascia rolling exercises is to relieve tension or trigger points through self-massage.

What you need: fascia roller

a) Begin by rolling one leg from the Achilles tendon up to the calf. If one-legged rolling is too painful, place both legs on the roller side by side and then complete the exercise.

Scan the calf for painful spots by applying gentle pressure as you roll the inside and outside of the calf. Do this exercise for approx. 60 seconds.

To intensify the effect, cross your legs one on top of the other and then perform the exercise.

To intensify it even more, try to flex and point the foot when you identify a painful spot, and subsequently also flex and point the toes along with the foot.

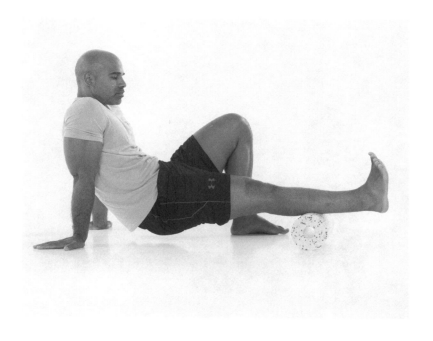

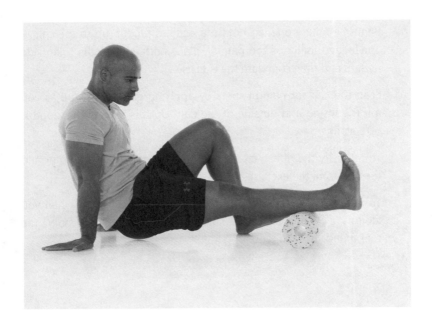

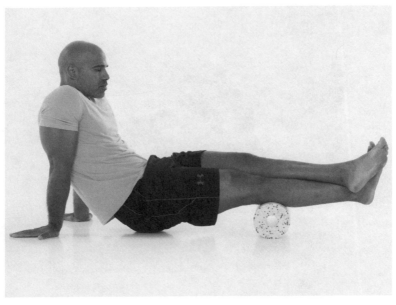

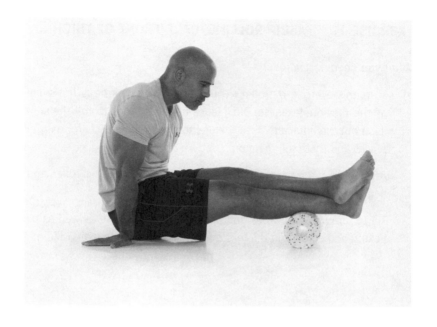

EXERCISE 12 – FASCIA ROLLING/CALF/FRONT OF THIGH

What you need: fascia roller

a) Start this exercise by rolling your shin. The technique is the same as the previous exercise. But please be careful not to roll the shin itself but the adjacent muscle. Here, too, scan the muscle for painful places and try to roll them out.

After rolling the shin muscle, place your thigh on the roller and begin to roll out the muscle at the front of the thigh.

Try to integrate your toes and ankle into this exercise as well as by flexing and extending the toes and ankle of the leg you are rolling.

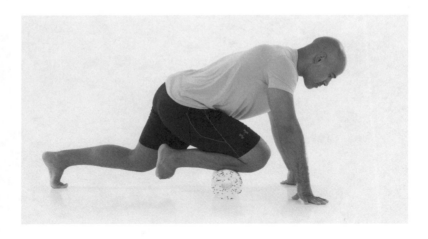

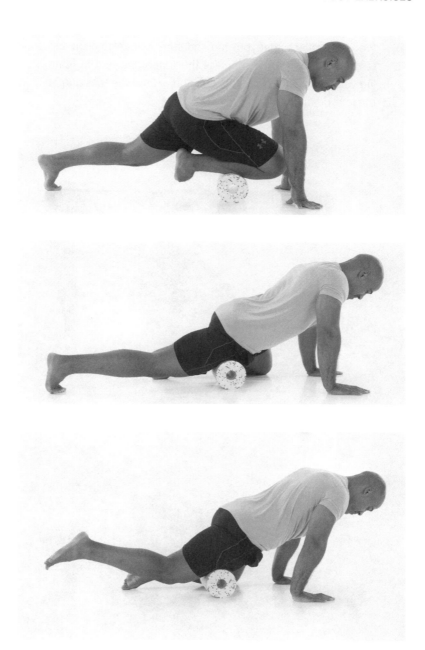

b) Place the roller under your hip and start rolling from the hip down to the knee. As you do so, place the supporting foot in front of the leg you are rolling. Here, too, flex and extend the toes and ankle of the leg you are rolling.

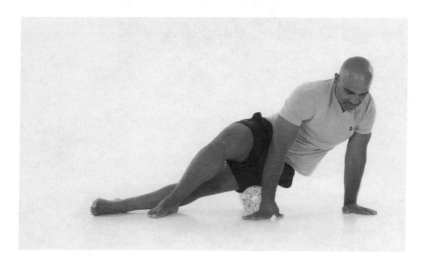

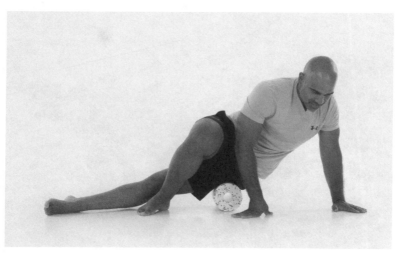

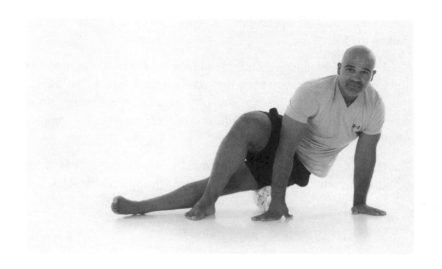

EXERCISE 14 – INCLINE BOARD/STABILITY

This exercise practices barefoot walking on different surfaces. What matters here is simply that you walk barefoot outside on round pebbles, gravel, and finally sharp little stones. In doing so, the degree of difficulty gradually increases. You can do this exercise outside anywhere. For example, you can walk on a pebble path in front of your house or on a gravel path in the forest.

You begin by just standing on these surfaces in a wide stance, since the stimulus is already quite intense and your soles will need to get used to this unfamiliar surface. The next step is to stand on the different surfaces on one leg so that your weight shifts and further intensifies the stimulus. Finally, walk carefully on the surfaces.

The purpose of this exercise is to activate the sensory motor skills of the soles (proprioception). This improves sensory perception of the soles.

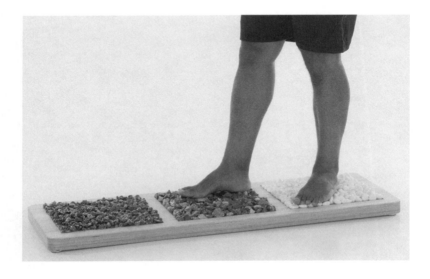

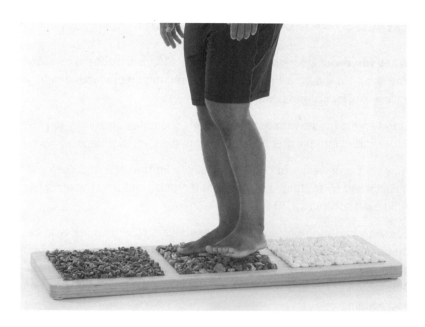

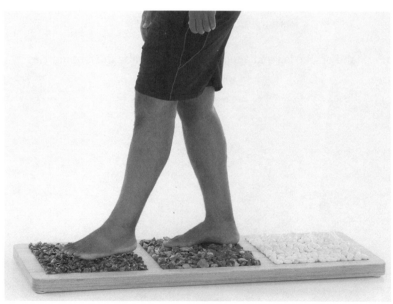

EXERCISE 14 – INCLINE BOARD/STABILITY

What you need: create or build a slanted surface that doesn't wobble. You should stand on a firm surface. This situation reproduces a natural incline like, for instance, on a hillside.

Stand on the incline with both legs, slowly straighten up and try to press your big toes into the ground or rather into the slanted surface.

Now shift your weight to one leg and slowly lift the other leg. Keep your balance and try to stand upright. First lift one leg and then the other leg. Hold each position for 20 seconds.

You activated the soles during the pre-exercise. Now the idea is to get the foot and ankle used to unfamiliar situations again, like pronation and supination. Here it is beneficial to get the foot used to the pressure during supination and teach the ankle how to deal with the situation appropriately.

Adjusting the incline to a steeper angle can intensify this exercise.

a)   Stand on one leg and alternate feet to stabilize the foot muscles.

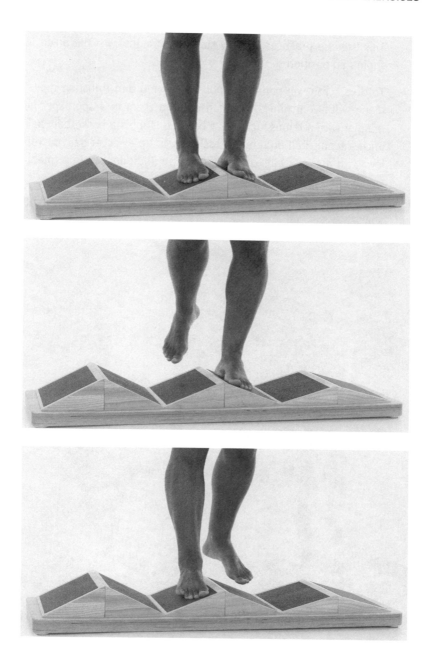

b) This exercise practices actively standing upright with the ankle in supinated position.

To do so, you will perform various balancing and thrusting movements with your hands. You can perform them in a sport-specific manner with a tennis racket or a ball: e.g. dribble a basketball, balance a tennis ball on a tennis racket, hold up a soccer ball, do volleys with a soccer ball, or squats with an additional weight (medicine ball).

The exercise execution is the same as the previous exercise. Begin by doing the variations in a wide stance, then on one leg.

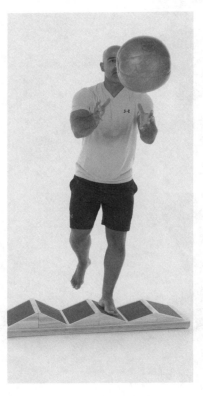
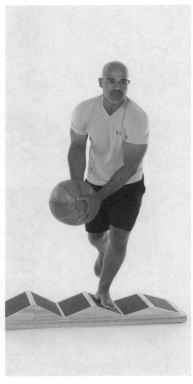

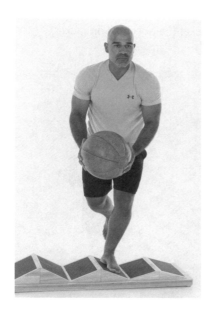

A different angle:

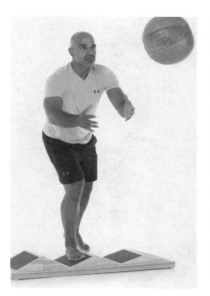
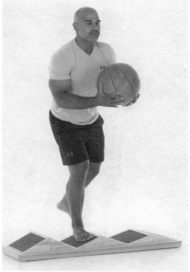

c) One-legged stance with tennis racket (balance ball on racket).

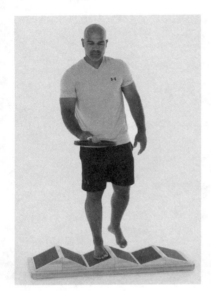
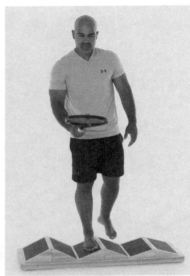

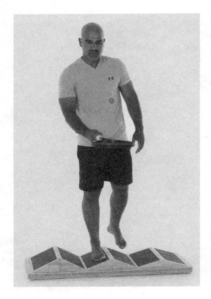
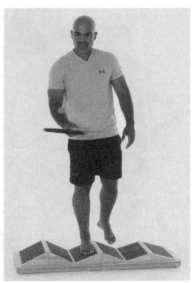

d) One-leg stand with basketball (bouncing).

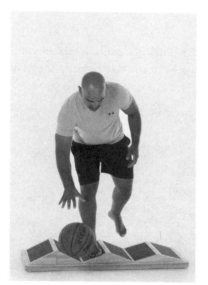
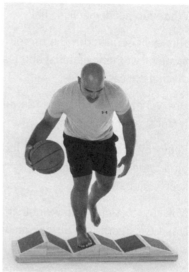

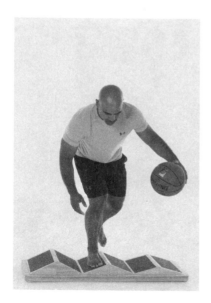
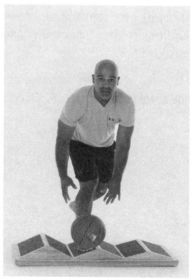

EXERCISE 15 – MOBILITY/STABILITY/LATERALITY

What you need: medicine ball

This exercise includes the use of leather medicine balls. Medicine balls made of synthetic material and plastic are not suitable because they slip much more easily.

One variation would be to use different sized medicine balls.

Begin by standing with each foot on a large medicine ball and try to keep your balance.

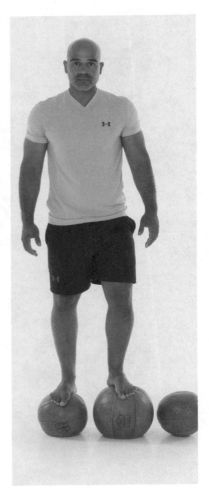

Now try to shift your weight and stand with both feet on one medicine ball.

You can increase the degree of difficulty of this exercise by decreasing the size of the standing surface by, for instance, standing on a smaller medicine ball.

Here, too, the sole is activated and the ankle becomes more flexible.

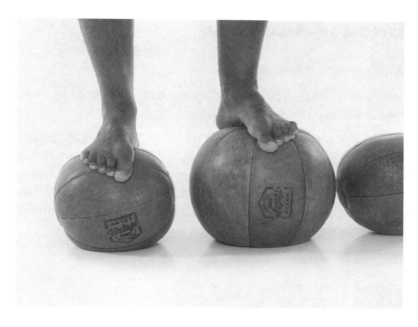

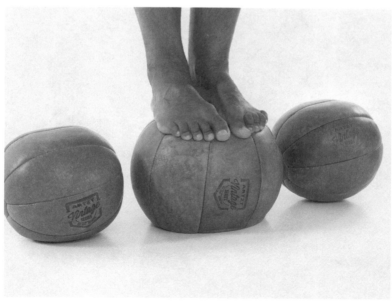

EXERCISE 16 – BALANCE BEAM

What you need: balance beam

This exercise is similar to the standing and walking exercises on an incline as well as on the medicine ball.

Varying the different surfaces works the sole's sensitivity and stability. First, you should learn to stand on a balance beam with both feet, find your balance, then do the exercise on one leg, and finally start moving by walking across the balance beam. Adding implements like a basketball or a medicine ball will work different movement patterns and increase the degree of difficulty.

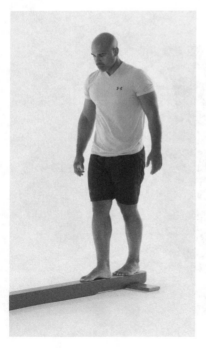 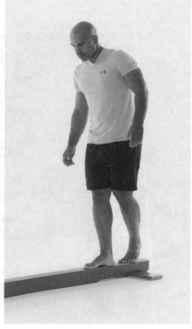

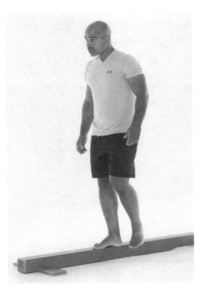
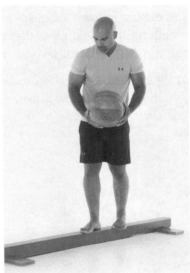
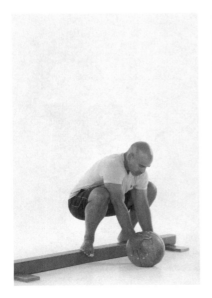
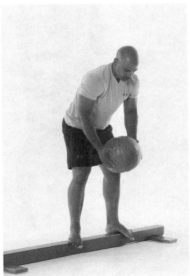

EXERCISE 17 – JUMPS

This exercise includes the use of a molded floor panel. This floor panel is a substitute for an extremely uneven surface and functions as an aid. You can also do this exercise on grass or on a forest floor, or even on a log.

a)   Jump onto the uneven surface with both legs. Jumping increases the overall load and activity. Here jumping represents the stress and strain of running.

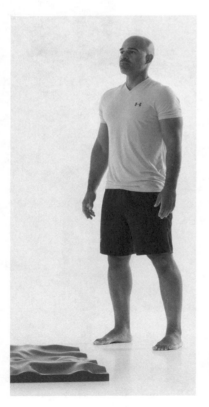
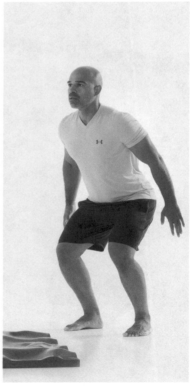

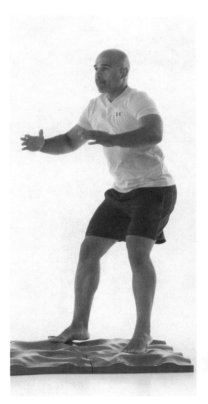 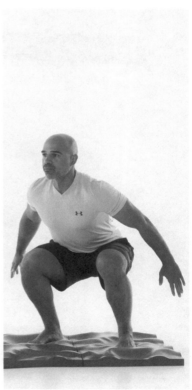

b) In this variation, you jump onto the uneven surface with just one leg.

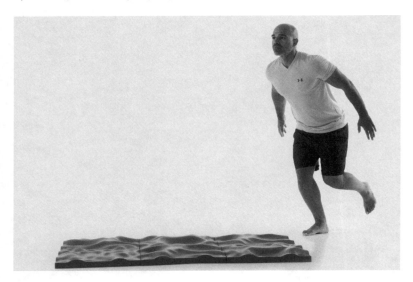

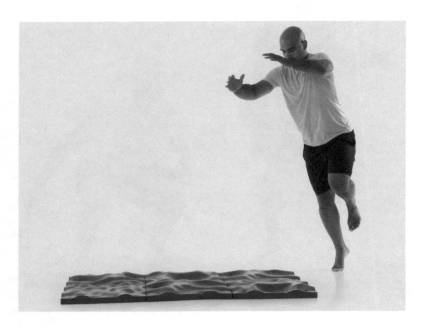

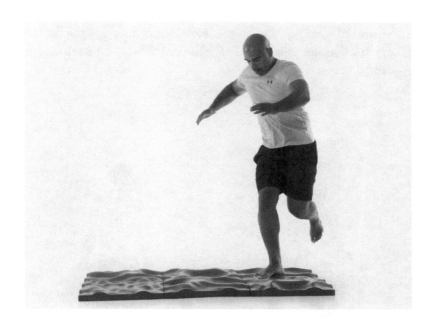

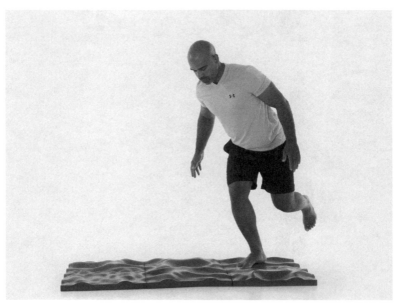

c) Begin by jumping rope on the level floor first. In addition to the jumps, you are using the rope as an aid to work on hand to eye coordination.

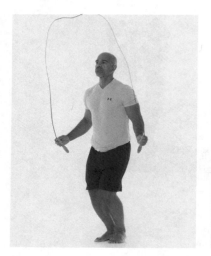
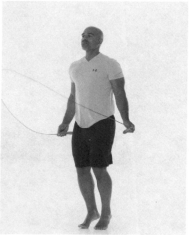

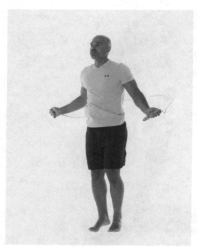

d) Now perform this exercise on the uneven surface, increasing the degree of difficulty.

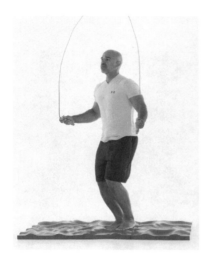
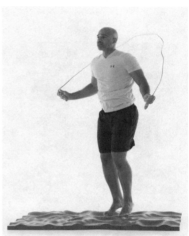

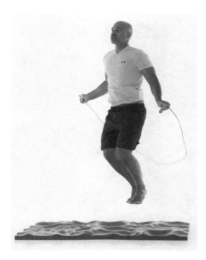

EXERCISE 18 - FOOT STRENGTH

What you need: loop band

a) Stretch the loop band between your two big toes and pull the toes apart. It is important that only the toes work. Your feet and legs should not move.

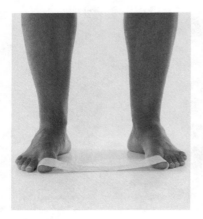
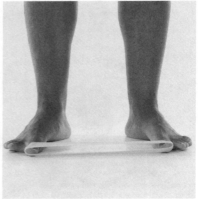

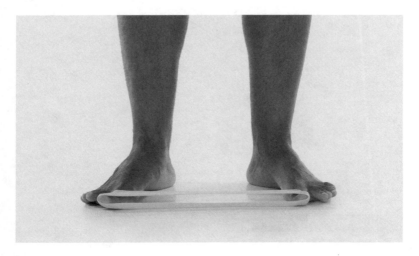

b) Place the loop band around one big toe and then add tension to the band with your hand.

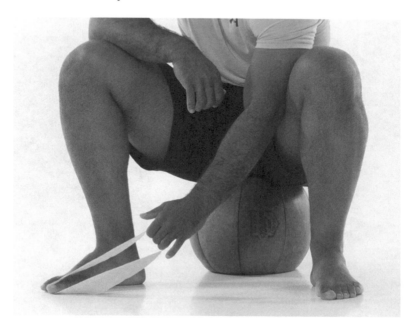

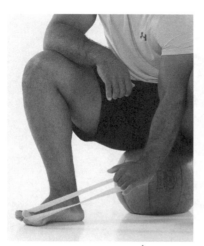
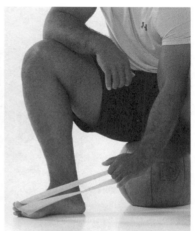

c) In this variation, you stretch the loop band around the entire foot and pull on it with your hand. Simultaneously rotate the foot to the outside against the band's resistance.

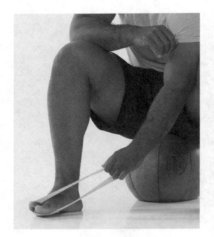 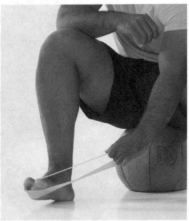

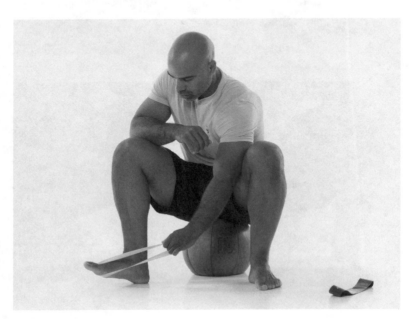

37 HELLO, FEET: GOOD MORNING WORKOUT

You may not have been aware of this, but when you start your day, it is your feet that take the lead and pave the way. After all, regardless of whether you like to sleep in or get up early, you explore the floor in front of your bed with your feet before your body moves into an upright position. It is how they start their day's work and carry you through the remainder of the day.

It therefore makes sense to prepare them for their job and appropriately gear them up for their daily burden.

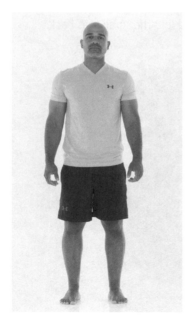

That's where a little Toebility workout is just the right thing. Begin by standing upright with your arms relaxed at your sides and toes pressing into the floor.

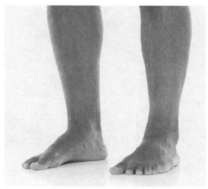

Now grip the floor with your big toe and lift the small toes.

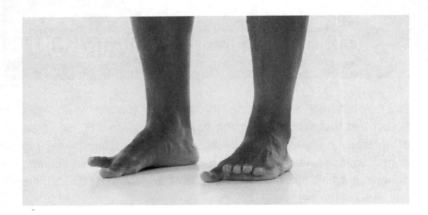

Next try to mobilize the metatarsophalangeal joint by standing on one leg and pressing the other foot into the floor, leading with the toes. As you do so, spread the big toe forward and fold the small toes back.

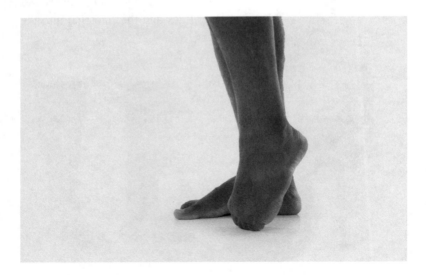

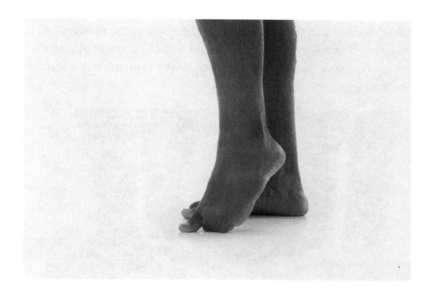

Now continue in the other direction. Fold the big toe back and let the small toes press forward.

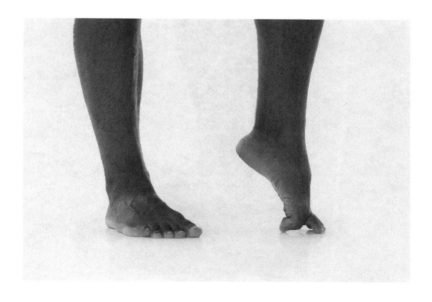

Close this unit with the caterpillar by again gripping the floor with all of your toes, and try to pull yourself forward with the strength of your toes. As an alternative, you can place a towel on the floor and pull it towards you with your toes.

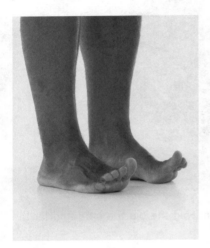 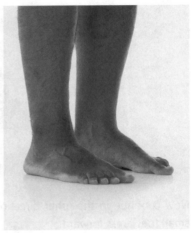

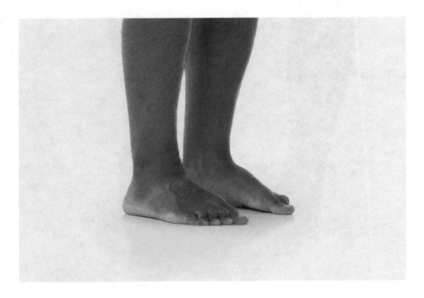

With a band:

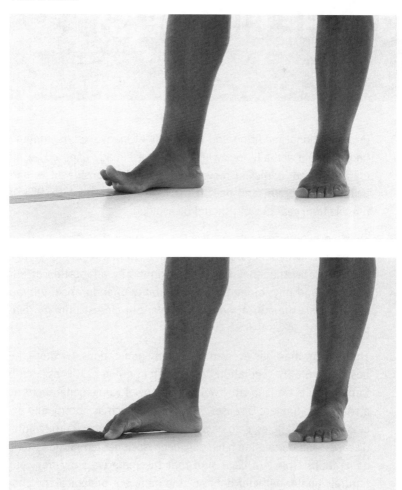

You have now activated and strengthened the sole of your foot and mobilized the joints in your toes. You have moved them through their range of motion.

You can find additional exercises in the large workout section.

38 THE BIG TOE(S)

1. In conventional medicine and the minds of many experts, running (most people actually jog, which we have already exposed as an unnatural and inefficient movement pattern) is considered as particularly dangerous, and due to the high injury rates (30-79% of runners from year to year) should be avoided.

2. From an evolutionary point of view, we know that humans have traveled long distances on foot for more than two million years. We also know that they have run upright. The adaptation of our anatomy and physiology to the vital ability of endurance running has given us the critical advantage over our closest primate relatives.

3. The modern man has evolved over many generations. Of those, he has spent 6,666 generations as a hunter-gatherer, 366 as a crop farmer, 7 as a working city dweller, and now 4 whole generations as a sitting zoo-human. Diseases of civilization such as obesity and excess weight, diabetes, cardio-vascular diseases, cancer, autoimmune diseases, and depression have only been documented in the last 11 generations. This is a clear sign that the more we stray from our natural "hunter-gatherer habitat," the more our biological, psychological, and social health suffer.

4. Due to the high occurrence of running injuries, these must also be included in the diseases of civilization. It is not just that we have developed into perfect long-distance runners, because this was something that we did before, barefoot on hard, rocky ground. In fact,

humans developed footwear like sandals or moccasins during the Later Stone Age over 40,000 years ago.

5. Upon closer examination and in the light of evolution, it is only logical that humans have adapted very well to their species-specific forms of movement, walking and running, barefoot or rather without modern athletic shoes. Current research on our biomechanics supports this logic with data. The technique similar to that of an experienced barefoot runner (effective forefoot strike and shorter strides) can significantly reduce the stress and strain and minimize the risk of injury.

6. The science behind barefoot running is indisputable. The problem is the practical application of the science so that it has a positive effect on modern shoe-wearing man. Learning a competent barefoot runner's technique is relatively easy. The kinematics, the forms of movement of a competent barefoot runner, can be taught with modern teaching principles and methods, and biofeedback tools like video analysis.

7. The foot itself is a slightly bigger challenge. People who habitually wear shoes no longer have a natural, aboriginal foot. Characteristics like weak muscles, a high stiff instep, shortened tendons, and crooked toes are not seen among naturally living people.

8. The reason is the habitual wearing of anatomically incorrect shoes since earliest childhood. The foot of a child consists largely of cartilage that turns completely to bone by age 18-19 in girls and age 20-21 in boys. During this time, the foot is very vulnerable and locked in hard and stiff footwear. The foot begins to adapt its structure to the shoe (Chinese foot binding effect). By contrast, the traditional footwear of hunters and gatherers was very soft and adaptable, and therefore adapted to the shape of the foot.

9. The advantages of barefoot running occur in combination with natural footwear. In my experience, the lack of natural functionality

of the foot and ankle is the main reason for why the adjustment to barefoot running can vary from 6 weeks to 2 years. It is also a very slow and painful process. The foot's hardware is subject to the same principles of training theory and adaptation as the rest of the body.

10. Our body possesses an incredible ability to adapt and heal. Nevertheless, too much training too soon will lead to an overload of the structures, coherently causing pain and injury. It is absolutely not advisable to throw away your shoes and just start running. Instead you should invest a couple of months and first practice standing and walking to allow proprioception and gravity to do their job.

So now the question is no longer whether running barefoot is natural, beneficial, or good for you, but whether you find the effort of adapting and training worth it. It is a decision much like that of parents-to-be deciding whether their newborn should be nursed at its mother's breast, or rather be fed with a synthetic industrial product from a bottle.

Whatever seems to be easier, the advantages of feeding a newborn mother's milk are scientifically, similarly undisputed.

REFERENCES

Adam, I. D., Gary, J., Geissler, F., Wang, J., Saretsky, Y., Daoud, A. & Lieberman, D. E. (2012). *Foot Strike and Injury Rates in Endurance Runners: A Retrospective Study.* Medicine & science in sports & excercise.

Bompa T. O. (1994). *Periodization: Theory and Methodology of training. Champaign: Human Kinetics.*

Bowerman, W. J. & Harris, W. E. (1979). *Jogging.* TBS.

Bramble, D. M., Lieberman D. E. (2004). *Endurance running and the evolution of Homo. Nature.* 432:345-352.

Carrera-Bastos, P., Fontes-Villalba, M., O´Keefe, J. H., Lindeberg, S. & Cordain, L. (2011). The western diet and lifestyle and diseases of civilization. *Research Reports in Clinical Cardiology.*

Earls, J. (2016). *Born Walk.* Aachen: Meyer & Meyer.

Hodges N. & Williams M. A. (2012). *Skill Acquisition in Sport: Research, theory and practice.* Westborough: Taylor & Francis Ltd.

Hoffmann, P. (1905). The feet of barefooted and shoe-wearing peoples conclusions drawn from a comparative study. *J Bone Joint Surg Am.;* s2-3:105-136.

Lieberman, D. E., Bramble, D. M., Raichlen, D. A. & Shea, J. J. (2006). *Brains, Brawn, and the Evolution of Human Endurance Running Capabilities The First Humans-Origin and Early Evolution of the Genus Homo.*

Lieberman D. E., Venkadesan M., Werbel W. A., Daoud A. I., D'Andrea

S., Davis I. S., Mangeni R. O. & Pitsiladis Y. (2010). Foot strike patterns and collision forces in habitually barefoot versus shod runners. *Nature.* 463:531-535.

McDougall, C. (2015). *Born to Run: Ein vergessenes Volk und das Geheimnis der besten und glücklichsten Läufer der Welt.* München: Heyne.

Morton J. D. (1948). *The human foot: Its Evolution, Physiology and Functional Disorders* New York: Columbia University Press.

Robbins, S. E. & Hanna, A. M. (1987). Running-related injury prevention through barefoot adaptations. *Med. Sci. Sports Exerc.* 19, 148–156.

Taunton, J. E., Ryan, M. B., Clement, D. B., McKenzie, D. C., Lloyd-Smith, D. R. & Zumbo, B. D. (2003). A prospective study of running injuries: the Vancouver Sun Run „In Training" clinics. *Br J Sports Med. 37*:239-44.

Trinkhaus, E. & Hong Shang, A. (2008). Anatomical evidence for the antiquity of human footwear: Tianyuan and Sunghir *Journal of Archaeological Science* 35.

Surgeon General's Call to Action to Support Breastfeeding (2011). US department of Health and Human Services.

van Gent, R. M., Siem, D., van Middlekoop, M., van Os, A. G., Bierma-Zeinstra, A. M. A., Koes, B. W. (2007). Incidence and determinants of lower extremity running injuries in long distance runners: a systematic review. *Br. J. Sports Med.* 41, 469-4807.

van Mechelen W. (1992). Running injuries. A review of the epidemiological literature. *Sports Med.* 14:320-335.

Wolff, J. (1891). *Das Gesetz der Transformation der Knochen.* Berlin: A. Hirschwald.

CREDITS

Photos

Cover photo: ©five Konzept GmbH & Co. KG

Exercise photos: Mira Hampel, www.mirahampel.de

All other photos: pp. 69, 88, 89: ©Ralf Kälin; 81, 94, 96: ©AdobeStock

Illustrations (inside and cover): Maike Maier, www.macamoca.de

Cover and interior design: Annika Naas

Typesetting: ZeroSoft

Managing editor: Elizabeth Evans

Copyeditor: Qurratulain Zaheer

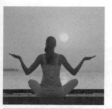
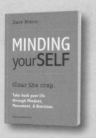
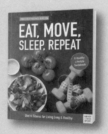

FROM MEYER & MEYER SPORT

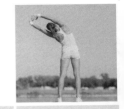

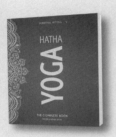

Paperback, 8.3 x 10"
424 pp., in color
983 photos + illus.
ISBN: 9781782551850
$34.95 US

Martina Mittag

HATHA YOGA
THE COMPLETE BOOK

Hatha Yoga is the most complete training book on hatha yoga. The 34 various flows and progressions are suitable for both yoga instructors and practitioners. For those looking for the best resource on hatha yoga, this book is a must.

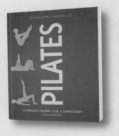

Paperback, 8.3 x 10"
384 pp., in color
1039 photos + illus.
ISBN: 9781782551867
$29.95 US

Rahn/Lutz

PILATES
COMPLETE TRAINING FOR A
SUPPLE BODY

Pilates provides comprehensive knowledge and contains a variety of exercises as well as professional tips and hints that will help to strengthen the body's core and supporting muscles.

MEYER & MEYER Sport
Von-Coels-Str. 390
52080 Aachen
Germany

Phone   +49 02 41 - 9 58 10 - 13
Fax   +49 02 41 - 9 58 10 - 10
E-Mail   sales@m-m-sports.com
Website   www.m-m-sports.com

MEYER
& MEYER
SPORT